Healthy Sexuality Development

A Guide for Early Childhood Educators and Families

Healthy Sexuality Development

A Guide for Early Childhood Educators and Families

Kent Chrisman and Donna Couchenour

An NAEYC Comprehensive Membership Benefit

National Association for the Education of Young Children
Washington, D.C.

Photographs © by
Hildegard Adler: 21
CLEO: 52
Jean-Claude LeJeune: cover, 34, 43, 62
Jonathan A. Meyers: 24
Marilyn Nolt: 2

National Association for the Education of
   Young Children
1509 16th Street, NW
Washington, DC 20036-1426
202-232-8777 or 800-424-2460
www.naeyc.org

Through its publications program the National Association for the Education of Young Children (NAEYC) provides a forum for discussion of major issues and ideas in the early childhood field, with the hope of provoking thought and promoting professional growth. The views expressed or implied are not necessarily those of the Association. NAEYC thanks the authors, who donated much time and effort to develop this book as a contribution to the profession.

Library of Congress Control Number
   2002111542
ISBN 1-928896-05-7
NAEYC Product #221

Publications editor: Carol Copple
Copyediting: Mary Gawlick and Lacy Thompson
Editorial assistance: Natalie Cavanagh
Design and production: Malini Dominey

Printed in the United States of America

About the Authors

Kent Chrisman, Ed.D., is an associate professor in the early childhood program of the Department of Teacher Education at Shippensburg University in Pennsylvania. He is the former director of the Rowland School (prekindergarten through fifth grade) at Shippensburg University and the Early Childhood Laboratory (infants through first grade) of Stephen F. Austin State University in Texas. Kent coauthored the book *Families, Schools, and Communities: Together for Young Children*.

Donna Couchenour, Ph.D., is professor of early childhood education in the Department of Teacher Education at Shippensburg University. In her 25 years in early childhood education, she has been a Head Start teacher and director and the director of child development laboratories at Oklahoma State University and West Virginia University. Donna is coauthor of *Families, Schools, and Communities: Together for Young Children*.

Contents

Acknowledgments

Many people have made important contributions to this book. We appreciate those teachers, families, and students in early childhood teacher preparation who have been willing to consider the sensitive and sometimes controversial topic of healthy sexuality development in young children.

Of particular note is the work of Amy Gottshall and Tricia Koons. Their efforts in undergraduate research at Shippensburg University and at conference presentations both locally and nationally added an important dimension to this project. Stacey Horschler was an invaluable and dedicated graduate research assistant during the early stages of this work.

Conference participants at local, national, and international meetings provided a great deal of support in terms of suggested resources and affirmed the need for this kind of book. We have been overwhelmed by the substantial interest in this topic. This continuous affirmation led us to believe that a book on healthy sexuality development in young children was needed so early childhood teachers, administrators, and families with young children could gain access to the vast array of resources and information concerning best practices for supporting young children's healthy development.

Introduction

Basic Concepts in Healthy Sexuality Development

Two teachers engaged in conversation . . .

"Thank goodness I teach 3-year-olds. Disagreements about sexuality discussions in the classroom do not affect me!"

"Healthy sexuality development begins at birth. One of the first questions most people ask with the arrival of a new baby is . . ."

"Boy or girl? But that question is not meant to be sexual."

"I guess it depends on how you define sex, sexual, *and* sexuality. *Children are defined by their gender and are learning about sexuality from the day they are born. And it is up to the important adults in their lives to decide what and how children learn about sexuality. Adults will set the tone for values about sex."*

"So, parents and teachers of even very young children have responsibility for helping children to understand issues related to sex?"

"Yes. If children do not learn it from their parents and teachers, they will learn it somewhere else. And other sources such as the media and peer encounters may not provide important information for healthy sexuality development."

"But how do I know where to begin? I haven't had any training in this area. No one discussed this topic in my teacher preparation program. And personally, in my family we didn't mention the word sex *aloud."*

Healthy sexuality development begins at birth. From the day a child is born, many decisions are made that are related to the baby's gender. At birth and, many times, prenatally, children are identified as girls or boys. This identification is based solely on the child's genitalia. When medical staff and families observe a vulva, they announce a baby girl; when they observe a penis and testicles, they proclaim a boy. After this pronouncement, a name is selected that denotes the child's gender in most societies. Clothing, color choices, decorations, and toys are often purchased with the child's gender in mind. All of these selections are based on nothing but the child's genitals.

Information in this booklet is based on several premises:

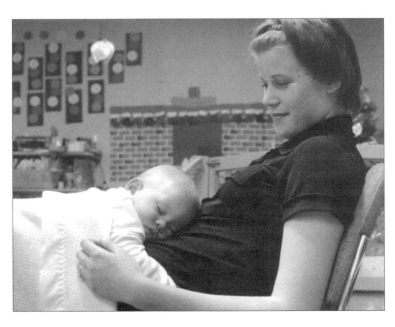

- Healthy sexuality development begins at birth.

- Children learn about sexuality the same way they learn about everything else— through words, actions, interactions, and relationships.

- Families are children's primary teachers about sexuality development.

- Early childhood teachers and administrators support children's healthy sexuality development both directly, as they interact with children, and indirectly, as they work with families and plan programs.

Infants must be given sensitive, responsive nurturing from their primary caregivers so they learn to trust that the world is pleasing (Erikson 1968). This sense of trust or

Healthy Sexuality Development

attachment is believed to be a critical emotional bond providing the foundation for the child's later ability to form positive relationships with others, including adults, siblings, and peers. Much of this same important adult-infant interaction that supports the baby's physical, cognitive, social, and emotional development also promotes healthy sexuality development. In fact, one way to understand sexuality development in young children is to relate it to all the developmental processes (Couchenour & Chrisman 2000b).

Children learn about sexuality the same way they learn about everything else. They learn through words, exploration, play, interactions, and relationships. Many early childhood teachers and administrators have expertise in understanding how children learn and think. A great deal of both preservice and inservice professional development emphasizes children's cognitive development. Many early childhood teachers have observed infants' motor activity and their use of all five senses: seeing, hearing, smelling, tasting, and touching. The work of Jean Piaget ([1936] 1952) has informed us that this activity and use of the senses is how very young children acquire knowledge.

As children near the age of two, they begin to use symbols—language and pretend play—to understand their world. Because children are naturally curious about much of their world, they are also curious about their own and others' bodies. And because preschool children learn primarily through observation, exploration, and play, they sometimes carry over these ways of learning to their curiosity about bodies: showing their genitals to peers, touching body parts that are typically covered, and even engaging in sex play. It is important for adults to understand that just as children's thought processes are different than those of adults, child sexuality is also different than adult sexuality. Children's sexuality is different from adults' sexuality in at least three ways (Rothbaum, Grauer, & Rubin 1997).

1. Children are curious and playful. Adults have knowledge about sex and are responsible for their decisions and behavior. One preschooler learned that it may not be proper to discuss certain body parts after running through her living room filled with visitors immediately after having her bath, patting her bottom and saying, "This is my butt. Ha, ha, ha!"

2. Children are as spontaneous and open about sex as they are about anything else. Healthy adult sexuality is typically deliberate and private. A preschool teacher reported a bathroom discussion with one boy who announced, "Boys have penises and girls have vaginas. I'm a boy, and this is my penis."

3. Children may find the topic of sexuality at once exciting and disgusting, and they may imitate the sensuality of adult models in their lives. Because of cognitive and biological differences between children and adults, however, children lack the eroticism evident with adult sexuality. Preschoolers frequently incorporate spousal roles into their dramatic play. These roles often take on the social acts that children have observed, so although children speak about who they will marry, teachers and parents should be aware that young children generally lack the understanding that sexual intercourse is involved in marital relationships.

The role of families

Family members are the primary teachers for children's sexuality development (SIECUS Early Childhood Task Force 1998). Most children grow up in families. Even though family structures vary and some children belong to more than one family, this intimate environment is where children learn the most about how people care for one another in different ways. Most often, the adults who are parenting give children early information about sexuality, such as gender identity, names of body parts, words for toileting, and so on. Families share attitudes, beliefs, and values about sexuality that may come from their culture.

One attitude in the United States today is that young children do not need to know about sexuality. Unfortunately, when children's curiosity about sex is ignored or when children are told that they should not say "those words" or are shamed for asking questions, an attitude of secrecy is conveyed. In fact, young children learn something about sexuality from their families whether families intend for them to or not. For example, when parents behave secretively about sex, children learn that sex is a secret.

In some households, adults talk openly about sexuality and are comfortable with nudity within the home. In other families, adults maintain a greater degree of privacy and restraint with respect to sexual matters. Although both of these approaches will affect children's understanding of sexuality, neither one is, by itself, healthy or harmful. Families can demonstrate a wide variety of differences that all reflect positively on children's understanding. Elements common to families who support healthy sexuality development in children include respectful interactions with one another, appropriate expressions of affection among family members, and a sensitive awareness of both expected behaviors and unacceptable behaviors.

The role of educators

Early childhood teachers also support children's sexuality development both directly and indirectly. Direct support for children's healthy sexuality development occurs through teachers' interactions and conversations with children. Some early education programs include a planned sex education curriculum. Even when this planned curriculum is not taught, teachers of young children frequently respond to children's questions and behaviors. Their responsibility is to provide accurate information and positive guidance in ways that are developmentally appropriate for young children. Whichever approach early childhood programs take to support healthy sexuality in young children, the sensitive nature of this topic requires that families be informed of policies and procedures. Ideally this information would be communicated through a handbook and would include additional information and resources to support families in their role as their children's most important sexuality educators.

By providing support for families of children in their care, early childhood teachers and directors can have a positive effect on children's healthy sexuality development. Some parents may ask for information about this topic, particularly when a new baby is expected in a family. However, many families may be uncomfortable broaching the subject of sex with their children's teachers.

Because so many adults do not understand what is typical for young children with respect to sexual development and behavior, they may have an underlying concern that something is not "normal" and, thus, avoid asking for professional opinions. For this reason, early childhood teachers and directors should be knowledgeable about children's curiosity with respect to sexuality and should be prepared to provide sensitive and appropriate support for parents or other family members so families can fulfill their responsibilities as children's primary sexuality educators. (See Resources, beginning on p. 81, for a list of appropriate literature and media for families.)

In the past, both educators and family members have been uncomfortable discussing topics related to childhood sexuality. Now, a greater understanding of child development provides the basis for more openly and objectively dealing with these concerns. In addition, societal changes have created a greater need to respond to children's sexual curiosity and behaviors. Children today are exposed to a great deal more sexual content through the various media outlets—including movies, sitcoms, music, and the news—than was true in the past. Society is now less secret about sex. For these reasons, adults should increase their comfort level by obtaining accurate information.

The goal is not necessarily to provide new information to adults, as through a sex education curriculum for children, but to support teachers and families in ways that allow them to understand children's development and to respond to children's sexuality objectively (Ryan 2000). The purpose of this book is twofold: (1) to provide information to early childhood educators and family members about typical sexuality development in young children and (2) to supply them with strategies for supporting healthy sexuality development in young children.

1

Defining Healthy Sexuality

Defining and explaining healthy sexuality development in young children in a holistic, integrated way makes sense. A holistic approach to sexuality development relates aspects from each developmental process to sexuality. Narrow definitions—for example, a definition of sex that restricts meaning to only sexual behavior—are too limiting when examining developmental processes. A developmental view acknowledges that behavior is affected by knowledge, understanding, attitudes, values, and other contextual influences. In this book, the importance of considering the whole child is the basic conceptual framework. Adults' actions and responses related to the sexual dimension of children's lives and development must always take into account children's capabilities and development in the physical (or motor), cognitive, social, and emotional domains.

So how might a teacher answer a preschooler's question, "What is sex, anyway?" Although one could answer this question in many acceptable ways, the recommended way to begin is by considering the context in which it was asked; that is, the sensitive adult would note anything in the environment that might have led to the child's question. A sensitive response would also take into consideration the differences between children's and adult's sexuality as explained earlier. A wise approach would be to check one's understanding of the child's question by asking what they think or what they have already heard about sex. Responses to a child's questions should be honest and, at the same time, not be more detailed than the child wants or needs (Wilson 1991).

Understanding the whole child

The following sections help us to better understand children's sexuality development in the context of the whole child by examining physical, cognitive, social, and emotional development. Understanding these developmental processes should help adults respond appropriately in many situations.

Physical development

Physical development refers to the child's physical growth, gross and fine motor skill development, coordination, and increasing control over bodily functions. One infant caregiver tells about an incident during a parent program on the current implications of the research on brain development that provides an example of how issues related to physical and sexuality development can overlap. After showing parents a videotape, the caregiver led a discussion during which one father expressed concern about the infant

massage techniques that were demonstrated. He said that he would not be comfortable touching his baby in that way. The caregiver asked the group of parents for more feedback and discovered that many of them connected massaging bodies with adult sexual behavior.

Because this caregiver understood the importance of touch for optimal brain development, her goal was to encourage greater amounts of touch and to help parents get beyond their discomfort. She asked some of the parents to tell how they already hold and touch their babies and suggested ways they might increase the level of touch with which they were comfortable. This caregiver was sensitive to the parents' concern about sexuality issues and suggested that, at future meetings, they could share common concerns that parents have about sex and obtain information to support healthy sexuality development in children. This topic led to a coordinated program that involved many families. The director invited experts from the fields of child development, human sexuality, and pediatrics. Among the resources that informed the discussions, the work of Tiffany Field, director of the Touch Research Institute, and Stanley Greenspan, clinical professor of psychiatry and behavioral sciences at George Washington University, contributed greatly.

Since the mid-1980s, Tiffany Field's research has demonstrated the positive effects of infant massage not only on babies' overall health, including weight gain and increased activity level, but also in increasing scores on a variety of developmental tests (Field 1998). Field has demonstrated effectiveness of massage on a variety of at-risk infants: preterm infants, those exposed prenatally to cocaine, and those born to HIV-positive mothers as well as to depressed mothers. In addition, massage has been effective with children who have arthritis, asthma, autism, and post-traumatic stress. Field is also studying the amount of touch that children receive in school settings (Santrock 2001).

Stanley Greenspan's model, based on knowledge of early cognitive and emotional development, stresses the importance of healthy and nurturing interactions between young children and the important adults in their lives (Greenspan 1990). The next three chapters describe more fully the kinds of interactions Greenspan describes as suited to the various periods in children's development.

Cognitive development

Cognitive development includes the changes that occur over time in a child's reasoning ability, problem-solving strategies, level of understanding, use of language and other symbols, memory, and motivation. Sophie, a pregnant kindergarten teacher attending a workshop on children's healthy sexuality development, explained her concern when children asked her how the baby got inside of her. The workshop participants shared a range of appropriate responses, including the following:

• The baby started from an egg that was already inside the mother.

• The baby was made when the dad's sperm joined the mother's egg.

• When the mother's egg and the dad's sperm got together, the baby began to grow.

Nearly all of the participants agreed that it would be important for the teacher to share with families that this topic was of great interest to the children. The teacher could also arrange parent education meetings or provide print resources to help families find appropriate ways to discuss this topic with their kindergartners. An excellent video resource to use in parent education meetings or to check out to families is *Raising Sexually Healthy Children* (Schrank & Hoke 1998).

Social development

Social development involves the child's ability to get along with others, develop friendships, establish identity, and understand right from wrong. At age 4, peers become very important. One way that children at this age can get the attention of other children is by using what teachers often call "toilet talk."

Jack, a preschool teacher, tells the story of one preschooler who, during free-play time, zipped through the entire classroom repeating, "Poopy, poopy, poopy." Soon children at every activity center were echoing "poopy" and laughing uproariously. Although Jack's previous experience had taught him that this activity was common social behavior for preschool children, he wanted to teach the children about more appropriate public behavior. So he talked to the director of the program, and together they decided to plan curriculum projects around the digestive system using a scientific point of view.

Jack found that even though some giggles were obvious at various times, he was able to take the mystique out of the word *poopy* by putting it in a biological context. The premise that every breathing, eating creature digests and excretes food to survive was a successful way to redirect children's thinking. In planning the curriculum for this topic, Jack found the books *Everyone Poops,* by Taro Gomi (1993), and *The Gas We Pass: The Story of Farts,* by Shinta Cho (1994), to be useful. Additional books, including *I Know Where My Food Goes,* by Jacqui Maynard (1999), *What Happens to a Hamburger?* by Paul Showers (1999), and *Look Inside Your Body*, by Gina Ingoglia (1989), also were incorporated into his planning. Further, Jack sent a letter to parents explaining the children's interest in this subject and his attempts to handle the interest through a study in biology.

Although the digestive system is separate from the reproductive system, children's interest in their bodies and bodily functions, especially those that involve the genital area, often poses challenges to parents and teachers of young children. Children's interest in genitals is especially challenging because adults must differentiate the elimination functions and the reproduction functions of the same body parts. Thus, it is important to address elimination language *and* reproduction language with children. (Ways to respond to "sex talk" are discussed further in Chapter 4.)

Adults who maintain a calm, caring approach as they respond to children's sexual curiosity help to promote healthy sexuality development and social competence. When families and educators understand the ways in which children's sexuality differs from adults' sexuality, they can more easily avoid overreacting to or ignoring behaviors that require a response or correction. Reacting in extreme ways and ignoring aggressive behaviors with sexual content are likely to lead to serious negative outcomes in children, including a loss of self-esteem, misinformation, feelings of guilt without understanding why, and unhealthy sexuality development (Kostelnik et al. 1998).

Emotional development

Emotional development comprises a child's ability to understand herself or himself, self-esteem, expression of emotions, and appropriate demonstrations of affection. Before children reach kindergarten age, they often have identified traditionally gender-related activities and toys and often choose to play only with children of the same gender.

Mr. Zane, a first-grade teacher, told about a girl in his class, Zoë, who came to school with a very special toy her mother had gotten for her over the weekend. When this male teacher asked the child where she got it, adding that he would like to have one, she said, "Oh, Mr. Z, these are only for girls." Expanding children's understanding of gender roles is an ongoing task for teachers.

Although it is important for children to develop a strong sense of self and incorporate what it means to be a girl or a boy, adults must help children to see that neither girls nor boys should be limited by gender roles. A teacher might ask Zoë why she believes that this toy is only for girls. Approaches that use stories or scenarios with puppets or props often help older preschool or primary-age children to better understand how boys and girls may play with the same toys and have the same interests. Some important reasons for assisting children in this understanding include the following:

• **Strict gender roles can limit friendships**. When Zoë is playing with her special toy, she is likely to deny boys access to it simply because she mistakenly thinks that only girls can play with that toy.

• **Strict gender roles can affect our feelings about ourselves.** Zoë is likely to believe that, if her toy is only for girls, then some other toys are only for boys. She will refrain from playing with these toys and, perhaps, will miss out on some area of competence or interest.

• **Strict gender roles can promote homophobia, and homophobia can promote the supporting of strict gender roles.** Zoë may get the message that boys who want to play with her toy are probably gay and that she should be wary of homosexuality (Cyprian 1998).

When children experience high levels of stress or boredom, they commonly turn to various sensory comforters. Some children may suck their thumbs, twirl a strand of hair, hug a particular stuffed animal, or rub a blanket. Some children hold or rub their genitals as a means of stress reduction (Briggs 1970). Adults may need to sometimes remind a few children that masturbation is not public behavior, but they must at the same time investigate possible stressors in a child's life and be sure that the child has access to satisfy-

ing friendships, healthy self-images, sensitive nurturing, and opportunities to engage in a variety of interesting activities.

The box that follows on the next page summarizes the areas of development discussed in this chapter. This summary underscores, once again, the interrelatedness of sexuality with all areas of human development.

Distinguishing staff education relating to healthy sexuality from information relating to child abuse

Workshops on child sexual abuse are essential for caregivers in early childhood programs. Child sexual abuse is perpetrated by unhealthy adults, and attentive caregivers play a key role in child abuse prevention. Early childhood professionals must contact their local child protective services agency in all cases of suspected abuse. The National Clearinghouse on Child Abuse and Neglect Information provides a list of toll-free numbers for reporting suspected abuse on their Website www.calib.com/nccanch/report.cfm or by calling them at 800-422-4453. Most reporting may be

A Young Child's Healthy Sexuality Development Relates to All Areas of Development

Physical development and behavior

Is interested in and explores body parts

Gains control over body functions

Experiences changes in the body as he or she grows older

Touches genitals or masturbates

Cognitive development

Learns about body parts and functions

Understands self as boy or girl

Understands others as girls, women, boys, or men

Is curious about and understands concepts about reproduction and other biological systems

Understands similarities and differences among humans

Social development

Is nurtured by loving adults

Makes friendships

Classifies behaviors according to gender roles

Develops basic awareness of morality

Responds to limits set by adults

Demonstrates assertiveness

Emotional development

Displays self-esteem and awareness of gender identity

Expresses affection and caring

Shows empathy

Shows respect for others

Manages anger, sadness, and joy appropriately

done anonymously. The emphasis in the present book is on supporting children's healthy sexuality.

An understanding of this healthy development encompasses a very different knowledge base. The study of healthy sexuality development in young children is, however, rarely part of preservice teacher preparation or staff training. The omission is not understandable if one views sexuality development in the context of typical child development. Staff development workshops could include topics such as responding to questions from children, use of correct anatomical labels, and strategies for redirecting inappropriate words or actions.

In part because of a prevalent attitude in society that leads adults to be ill at ease and unprepared to respond objectively to children's sexual curiosity and behaviors, very little specific research has been done in this area. Even with a dearth of scientific information, a great deal of "anecdotal information from teachers and caregivers supported a hypothesis that professionals who work with children often observed sexual activities which made them uncomfortable and which they believed were problematic" (Ryan 2000, 37).

Staff members and a group of multidisciplinary professionals at the Kempe Children's Center have worked since the early 1980s to develop an abuse prevention program for training professionals who work with children (Ryan 2000). A major emphasis in this project has been to use existing research to discover and affirm those sexual behaviors that are developmentally expected in children from birth through adolescence.

Teachers need such information on what child behaviors are within the range of typical development and what behaviors are not. Sometimes even a single occurrence of a behavior is a warning sign of possible child abuse or some other severe problem. When such a behavior involves one or more other children, there is likely to be an additional source of concern (Wardle 1998). Teachers must be sensitive to all children involved and document information carefully to provide for effective and caring follow-up. Wardle lists some of these unhealthy behaviors:

• Compliance in accepting intrusive and/or painful activity by another child
• Engaging in self-inflicted painful sexual activity
• Engaging in oral/genital contact with another child

• Engaging in simulated/attempted/completed intercourse while undressed
• Penetration of a girl's vagina with an object or finger
• *Forced* penetration of any orifice in a child (Emphasis added) (1998, 3)

These child behaviors differ from those that demonstrate healthy curiosity about sexuality because they may contain aggressive sexual actions (or a young child's compliance with these actions) that are not typical for young children. Through careful observation, teachers can differentiate among those interactions that are expected and those that may require reports of suspected child abuse. When teachers understand what to expect from children who have a healthy interest in sexuality, they can more clearly determine when children's behaviors need intervention and referral.

One group working on the children's sexuality project at the Kempe Center conducted a survey of elementary teachers. Teachers responded to anonymous questionnaires about the kinds of sexual behaviors they observed, the frequency of those behaviors, the competence the teachers felt they had in these matters, and whether or not the teachers had gone through academic preparation that focused on children's healthy sexuality development (Ryan 2000). Although every teacher reported a wide variety of sexual behaviors among children, most admitted that they often did not respond to those situations or that they redirected children or prohibited the behaviors. This study supported the project staff's hypothesis that teachers "observe a wide range of sexual behavior . . . and that they rarely had an objective basis for, or felt empowered to, respond to those behaviors in a meaningfully relevant fashion" (Ryan 2000, 39).

Relating healthy sexuality to developmentally appropriate practice

Some early childhood teachers seem to doubt the need to include information about healthy sexuality development in early childhood education. Some of the obstacles to preparing early childhood teachers for supporting children's healthy sexuality development include emotional discomfort, issues surrounding sex education in the schools, and problems defining the roles of families. However, an examination of several essential aspects of developmentally appropriate practices (Bredekamp & Copple 1997) provides support to the contention that this topic is highly relevant to quality early education. These essential aspects include the following:

• Intellectual and academic integrity

• Teacher-child interaction

• Effective and appropriate guidance

• Antibias endeavors and family involvement

Intellectual and academic integrity

In this area as in all others, early childhood teachers should include topics in the curriculum that reflect academic integrity. Children are curious about their own bodies and about how they came into the world. Topics about bodies and reproduction are of high interest and comprise information that is both scientific and social in nature. A common theme in early childhood programs is "All about Me" in which children provide materials such as photos and memorabilia for a bulletin board, construct booklets, and introduce family members. We know the importance of enabling children to understand what it takes to achieve a healthy body (good nutrition, exercise, preventive medical care, cleanliness, and rest).

In discussions about bodies, young children frequently ask questions or make comments for which teachers do not plan. When the comments touch on sexuality, many teachers admit ignoring the comments or redirecting children without providing information. Typically, however, these same teachers also understand that developmentally appropriate practices require sensitive responses to children's questions or comments with respect to any issue.

Ideally, teachers should expect and plan for children's comments, questions, and behaviors that indicate an interest in sexuality. Although many teachers get excited about children's thinking when it extends the topic at hand (e.g., the child who is experimenting with paint colors when mixing red and blue "discovers" purple), few adults react with the same enthusiasm when children announce details about their anatomy. In those situations, grown-ups would be more comfortable if children practiced discretion. However, because children's sexuality is typically spontaneous and open, curious and playful—

different from adults (Rothbaum, Grauer, & Rubin 1997)—discretion is not an appropriate developmental expectation for toddlers, preschoolers, or even children in primary grades.

Teacher-child interaction

The second aspect of developmentally appropriate practice has to do with teachers providing a model for respectful interaction with children. According to best practice in early education, teachers respond positively to children's curiosity and give additional information or affirmation to support children's thinking and understanding. When teachers ignore or reprimand children for words or behaviors that demonstrate inquisitiveness, especially inquisitiveness related to bodies and reproduction, then children may believe that they are wrong or bad to be interested in those topics. In contrast, sometimes teacher silence in response to children's comments may be interpreted as agreement. Although many teachers express discomfort or embarrassment when addressing children's expressions of sexuality, they have a professional responsibility to gain greater understanding of this aspect of child development, especially expected behaviors and those that are or may be troublesome. Teachers who overreact to some of these behaviors or who ignore them may inhibit the significant relationship between teacher and child.

Effective and appropriate guidance

A third area for appropriate practices relates to effective guidance strategies. When children engage in clearly inappropriate behavior such as touching another child's genitals or aggressively grabbing at another's body, teachers should use guidance strategies similar to what they would use with other behavior that needs to be stopped and redirected. Calm, matter-of-fact direction or redirection is often appropriate. For example, in a situation involving inappropriate touching, a teacher might start a discussion about what we can and should do with our hands, perhaps suggesting that hands are for helping others and ourselves. Teachers of young children make frequent use of techniques that redirect children to other activities or to other areas of the learning environment. Child behaviors that require a teacher response or correction are identified in Chapter 4.

Developmental Expectations	Recommended Practices
Infants and Toddlers	
Explore body parts, including genitals	Adults express healthy, accepting attitudes about children's bodies.
Develop positive or negative attitude about own body	Adults are attentive to infants during routines such as diaper changing and explain what is happening. Caregivers consistently respond to infants to keep them comfortable so they learn security.
Experience genital pleasure	Adults express healthy, accepting attitudes about children's body functions.
Encouragement to develop male or female identity	Adults praise accomplishments and help children to feel competent; parents are primary source of affection and care.
Learn expected behaviors by gender	Adults respect children's developing preferences as a healthy indicator of self-esteem; caregivers plan for active and quiet play for all children.
Preschoolers	
Aware of and curious about gender and body differences	Adults use children's natural curiosity to make sense of their world.
Masturbate unless taught not to	Adults facilitate the development of self-control, use redirection, and have expectations which match child's developing capabilities
Engage in various forms of sex play	Adults use redirection and have age-appropriate expectations of child's behavior; interactions are designed to promote positive self-esteem; adults design the play environment so supervision of children is possible at all times
Establish firm belief that they are either male or female	Adults facilitate opportunities to develop positive social skills; adults provide opportunities for children to gain understanding about themselves through observing and interacting with others.

Reprinted with permission from *Dimensions of Early Childhood*, Southern Early Childhood Association, www.SouthernEarlyChildhood.org.

Preschoolers (cont'd)

Enjoy bathroom humor	Adults use positive guidance techniques and have expectations which match child's development
Repeat curse words	Adults facilitate the development of self-control in children by using positive guidance such as modeling appropriate language.
Curious about from where they came	Adults use children's natural curiosity to make sense of their world; adults help children to understand themselves through interacting with other people

Kindergarten and Primary Children

Continue sex play and masturbation	Adults promote self-control through problem solving and redirection; adults try to prevent overstimulation and understimulation based on child's development; adults change activity centers frequently so children have new things to do
Curiosity about pregnancy and birth	Adults build on children's internal motivation to make sense of the world; teachers and parents are partners in the educational process.
Strong same-sex friendships	Adults facilitate the development of social skills at all times; adults ensure times with a close friend; adults model and expect acceptance and appreciation of differences and similarities
Strong interest in stereotyped gender roles	Adults plan and implement activities and materials to enrich the lives of all children
Have a basic sexual orientation	Adults view each child as a unique person; adults facilitate positive self-esteem
Choose gender-stereotypical activities	Adults provide a variety of activity choices, with children helping to select some topics; adults guide children's involvement in projects by extending their ideas and challenging their thinking.
Tease and call names	Adults promote prosocial behavior and facilitate the development of social skills; adults set clear limits and involve children in establishing rules for the classroom community or the home

Antibias endeavors and family involvement

Finally, teachers have opportunities to model and support tolerance, fairness, and respect for individual differences as they encourage children's healthy sexuality development. In addition to feeling general discomfort when dealing with issues involving sexuality and children, teachers also report that they are uncertain about which children's behaviors or ideas are acceptable and which are beyond an expected range (Rothbaum, Grauer, & Rubin 1997). Individual differences exist among children and families, differences that are influenced by the following factors:

• **Family communication with respect to sexuality.** Some children may come to the program knowing and using correct terms for body parts and understanding some information about reproduction; others may never have been exposed to these terms or to accurate information.

• **Family space for privacy.** Some children may be quite modest about their bodies, and others may not demonstrate much modesty, perspectives that are based partly on privacy expectations at home.

• **Media offerings available to children.** When children are exposed to sexuality that is inappropriate for their level of development, they may act out or ask questions that seem pseudomature.

• **Cultural variations.** Ongoing communication with families is critical to understanding values or perspectives that are important for cultural reasons.

• **Prejudices to which children are exposed.** Children are capable of learning homophobic and sexist responses at early ages.

• **Presence of older siblings.** Older siblings may use inappropriate words or discuss topics with sexual content without regard for the presence of younger children.

Because individual differences in behaviors can vary so greatly, early childhood teachers must maintain a high level of family involvement when contending with these issues in the classroom. Although many early childhood teachers may feel constrained by school policies with respect to sexuality development, they often can provide information for families to use with their young children at home and can ask families for information about their views and for their support in classrooms. The next three chapters of this book provide specific information for working with infants and toddlers, preschool children, and primary-age children. A summary for matching children's sexuality development with best teaching practice is found on pages 18–19.

Incorporating values into practice for supporting children's healthy sexuality development

Value statements used by the National Guidelines Task Force of the Sexuality Information and Education Council of the United States (SIECUS 1998) are included in this chapter because they are clearly stated; are consistent with best practice in early childhood settings; and can form the basis for parent discussions, staff training, and policy statements. SIECUS guidelines are based on a broad range of values related to human sexuality that are consistent with the beliefs of many communities within our pluralistic society. Every preschool and child care center should modify or adapt these values so they are consistent with

their community norms. Among the values expressed in the SIECUS guidelines, the following adaptations are relevant for preschool and child care centers to consider:

• Sexuality is a natural and healthy part of living that begins at birth and continues throughout life.

• All children should be loved and cared for and should feel safe and protected.

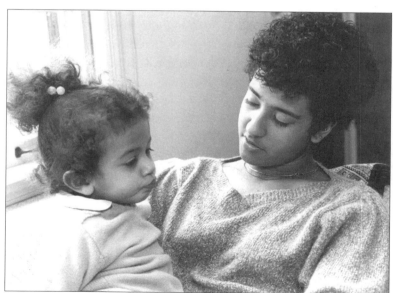

- All children should be respected and valued as unique individuals.
- Children experience their sexuality as a natural part of their development.
- Parents are their children's most important sexuality educators. The larger community of educators, early childhood staff, caregivers, and health professionals can also provide a positive influence in children's development toward sexual health.
- Children learn from how people touch them, talk with them, and expect them to behave as males or females. These messages children receive affect their future attitudes, values, and behaviors.
- Children are naturally curious about how their bodies look and work, about how male and female bodies differ, and about where babies come from.
- Children need to be helped to develop an awareness and appreciation of the human body and how it works.
- Children's understanding of sexuality is influenced by their parents, other family members, friends and neighbors, community, and school, as well as the media and other factors.
- Relationships should never be coercive or exploitative.

- Information about sex-related health risks and abuse should be presented to children within the context of positive information aimed at healthy personal and sexual development, such as human development and relationships, personal skills and health.
- In a pluralistic society like that of the United States, educators should respect the diversity of values and beliefs about sexuality that may exist in a community and among families.

✳   ✳   ✳

Early childhood teachers are often perplexed and uncertain about appropriate ways to respond to young children's expressions of sexuality. Gaining an understanding of which behaviors are expected and which are troublesome is a starting point for learning how to respond in appropriate and supportive ways. Working with families to assist in their understanding of healthy sexuality development in young children *and* to address their concerns and perspectives is an essential component of programs that support healthy sexuality development in young children.

2

Infants and Toddlers

The following three scenes are based on real-life experiences of parents, teachers, and caregivers of young children. In these cases all of the behaviors and concerns are related to typical sexuality development in children from birth to 3 years.

Pasha, mother of 6-month-old Robert, has been delighting in his rapid development. She eagerly shares with Nada and Lee, the infant caregivers at his child care center, all of his accomplishments, and the caregivers also update Pasha about their observations of Robert's development. This week, however, Robert has been touching his penis every time Pasha changes him and when she bathes him. Even though she is concerned about this behavior, she neither shares the information with Nada and Lee nor asks anyone else for information. She is not sure that Robert's behavior is normal, and she fears that, if she mentions it, someone might conclude she is a sexual abuser.

Frank, a teacher of toddlers in a child care center, has observed that Natasha masturbates throughout circle time. Janis, the assistant teacher, has also discussed with him that she has observed Natasha masturbating before she falls asleep at naptime. Frank is reluctant to discuss the sexual behavior with Natasha's mother, who is a single parent. Although Frank understands that it is not uncommon for toddlers to masturbate, the frequency of Natasha's masturbating concerns him. Further, as a male child care provider, he feels anxious about discussing a sexual issue with a single mom.

The East Side Child and Family Center is being renovated. A room for six 2-year-olds is one of the additions being made to the building. Sara, the center director, who has a great deal of training in early childhood education and 16 years experience, has suggested that one bathroom with three short toilets will be needed in the room. The board of directors and a few parents have expressed concern that the bathroom is too open, and some even believe that a separate area for boys and girls is necessary. Sara explains that the very young children can be better supervised and that staff can support toilet learning more effectively when dividers are not present in the bathroom.

Many adults, including both parents and educators, have not had opportunities to gain information about what to expect in terms of children's sexuality development. Even when adults do exhibit knowledge and understanding, such as in the case of the center director above, they are

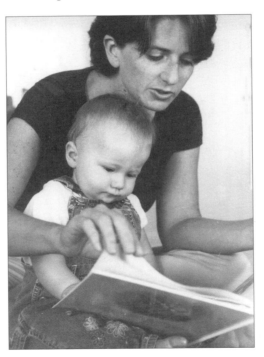

often questioned and criticized by those who operate within an adult framework of sexuality. One important function that an early childhood program can take on is to inform families about the differences between childhood and adult sexuality. Early childhood educators should communicate the differences between adult's sexuality and children's sexuality: Adults are knowing and aware of consequences whereas children are curious and playful; adults are self-conscious and desire privacy, and children are spontaneous and open; adults are motivated by eroticism, whereas children are superficial in their sensuality (their sensuality is not motivated by sexual desire and is often an imitation of observed adult behavior) (Rothbaum, Grauer, & Rubin 1997).

What a difference it would make to Pasha if she understood that, just as children discover their toes, they also discover their genitals. How unfortunate that our cultural taboos influence Frank's professional need to discuss a child's behavior with her parent. And how frustrating it is that so many adults project adult views of sexuality onto children.

Developmental understandings

Even among those adults who believe strongly in providing children with sex education, many would be surprised that, in fact, healthy sexuality development is a concern from birth. Parents and other primary caregivers of infants have a tremendous effect on children's very early views about their own bodies and bodily functions. "From the moment of birth, children begin to learn about love, touch, and relationships. Their experiences, impressions, and observations form the foundation of their future sexual attitudes and decisions" (SIECUS Early Childhood Task Force 1998, 1).

During these early years, children are likely to explore and express curiosity about all of their body parts. By age 3, many children are able to name various parts of their bodies. Some children have learned to ignore body parts that adults have taught them to consider as being private only, so they have no name for their genitals or for their posteriors. Other children have learned a variety of names such as "pee pee," "wee wee," "bottom," "privates," "pee-er," "peter," "butt," and "bum." Also, adults teach children a variety of informal terms for the bodily functions of urinating and defecating. These terms include "pee," "tinkle," "wee wee," "whiz," "poop," "poo poo," "potty," "make one," and "do a job." Interestingly, children learn "correct" terms for their eyes, ears, nose, mouth, teeth, hair, hands, feet, fingers, toes, knees, elbows, and so on.

Because very young children are interested in their own bodies as well as those of their friends and caregivers, these early years are very important for developing a positive or negative image of their own bodies. Adults who attentively explain what is happening to infants and toddlers during diaper changing, toilet learning, and bathing help to set a positive foundation for the child's healthy body image. Keeping young children clean and comfortable helps their bodies to feel good and increases their trust in others.

Physical development

• Infants are born with sexual organs.

• Boys may experience erections and girls may experience lubrication.

• Infants and toddlers explore body parts.

• Infants and toddlers typically experience pleasurable sensations when touching their own genitals.

• Infants and toddlers respond positively to healthy touches from loving adults.

• Toddlers begin the toilet learning process.

Cognitive development

• Infants' thinking is connected to all five senses and to their motor behavior.

• Toddlers begin to use symbols in their thinking, especially in pretend play.

• Infants and toddlers first are curious about their own bodies and then are curious about others' bodies; curiosity extends to genitals.

• Toddlers identify themselves as boy or girl and then identify others as boys or girls.

• Toddlers can learn to name body parts, including terms for male body parts such as scrotum, testicles, penis, and terms for female body parts, such as vulva, clitoris, and vagina.

• Toddlers observe differences in bathroom behavior for girls and boys.

• Toddlers increasingly use language for communication, including both appropriate words and inappropriate words.

• Toddlers increasingly make choices and decisions, primarily about food and playthings.

• Toddlers are learning how to solve problems and to get help when needed.

• Toddlers begin to acquire the ability to learn good hygienic practices: flushing, wiping themselves after toileting, and handwashing.

• Toddlers show greater energy and higher self-esteem when practicing healthy habits.

• Toddlers increase their understanding that elimination is natural for a healthy body.

• By the age of 2 years, toddlers understand that people differ (Derman-Sparks & the A.B.C. Task Force 1989).

Healthy Sexuality for Infants and Toddlers

- By the age of 2 years, toddlers can label peers correctly as boys or girls (Honig 2000).
- By the age of 3 years, toddlers can point out gender and racial differences (Derman-Sparks & the A.B.C. Task Force 1989).

Social development

- Infants and toddlers build trust as they experience positive interactions with loving adults.
- Infants respond to social interactions by gazing, smiling, vocalizing, and moving their bodies.
- Toddlers recognize primary caregivers and other people with whom they have frequent contact.
- For infants and toddlers, family structures are not all alike.
- Toddlers develop friendships.
- As early as the age of 3 years, gender differences exist in friendships (Maccoby 1998).
- When shown concern, caring, and kindness, infants and toddlers learn respect for others.
- Toddlers begin to use words to communicate with others and to resolve differences.
- Infants and toddlers receive different care and different messages based on gender.
- Toddlers begin to learn gender roles for the culture.

Emotional development

- Infants and toddlers need love, caring, and affection.
- Infants and toddlers are learning to receive and give love.
- Toddlers observe that demonstrations of affection differ according to relationships.
- Toddlers are learning ways to express emotions.
- Infants and toddlers learn to trust others to care for them.
- Toddlers learn to trust themselves as their skills increase.
- For infants and toddlers, trust is the basis for healthy self-esteem.
- Infants and toddlers are developing attitudes toward their own bodies.
- Toddlers are beginning to develop a male or female identity as defined by the context and culture (Maccoby 1998).

By age 3, many children can tell you, "I am a boy" or "I am a girl." However, few of them understand facts on which this sexual identity is based. Their information typically comes from parents who have provided the labels "girl" and "boy."

Children who are supported in their own play interests and styles are given a good beginning for healthy development. Adults who provide girls and boys alike both active and quiet play, as well as a variety of toys and materials, are setting the most optimal foundation for healthy sexuality development. The "Developmental Expectations" on pages 26–27 show indicators related to sexuality development in infants and toddlers for each developmental process.

Family members and teachers of children from birth to three 3 must be aware that, as they interact with young children, many of their behaviors and attitudes influence sexuality development. Caregivers who communicate positive regard for children's bodies and for their curiosity will contribute to healthy sexuality development. Adults who ignore or punish children's curiosity likely will influence children negatively.

Greenspan (1990) notes that, in very early infancy, the feelings of being soothed and comforted are likely babies' first experiences with pleasure. In coordination with these first experiences, the development of attachment begins; this emotional bond between adult and infant leads to "gleeful pleasure" (Greenspan 1990). As infants begin to be able to differentiate their sources of pleasure, at about 3 to 10 months of age, not only people but also bodily sensations become important to them. During this period, many infants learn that, when they touch their genitals, it feels good.

By the end of the first year or early in the second year, many infants initiate affectionate exchanges with parents and other important adults. They also continue to have a high interest in their bodies and curiosity about sexual differences between girls and boys. With an increase in cognitive capability and emotional growth, toddlers at about 2 years of age are able to internalize that their pleasure is associated with close relationships, warm interactions, and secure feelings. However, if parents or other important adults are withdrawn, aggressive, or intrusive, then those behaviors may become associated with

Healthy Sexuality Development

pleasure, which may lead to later maladaptive sexuality (Greenspan 1990).

Educator responsibilities for promoting healthy development in infants and toddlers include acceptance and celebration of all children, respect for individual differences, and appropriate expression of affection and feelings. Very young children need adult models for appropriate behavior and adults who will guide them to feeling good about themselves. In addition to providing responsive nurturing to infants and toddlers in their care, early childhood educators must also communicate with family members about the family's important role in supporting their children's healthy sexuality development.

Understanding how very young children think

The work of cognitive developmental theorist Jean Piaget ([1936] 1952) helps to explain the thinking of very young children. In the sensorimotor stage, from birth until about 2 years, children's thinking is tied directly to all five senses and to their motor behavior. Babies and toddlers increase their understanding as they interact with people and objects in their environment. In other words, babies must be active to think. For example, adults can perceive this form of infant cognition by watching babies as they play with a rattle or other toy. The following sequence is an example of cognitive development based on Piaget's theory (Piaget [1936] 1952):

1–4 months: Infant moves or vocalizes; the resulting sensations prompt the infant to repeat the action.

4–8 months: Infant shakes a toy and perceives a sound; action is repeated.

8–12 months: Infant sets out to cause the toy to make a sound, which marks the beginning of cause-and-effect understanding.

12–18 months: Child begins to use trial and error for problem solving.

18–24 months: Child begins to use symbols in thinking; now, he or she can think before acting (preoperational thinking), and imitation of others' behavior is possible.

By age 2, many toddlers are in Piaget's stage of preoperational thinking (Piaget [1936] 1952). The most important new ability children gain during this stage is the ability to use symbols more frequently in their thinking. In addition to being capable of imitating others, toddlers demonstrate the ability to use a concrete object to represent something else. Nevertheless, toddler thinking is markedly different from that of older children or adults. Piaget noted that children at this age have some common characteristics that affect their understanding. For example, toddlers are egocentric, meaning that they have difficulty understanding the perspective of another person. Curiosity about body differences may lead the toddler to some behaviors that concern adults: staring, asking questions, touching the genitals of another person. Although it is important for caring adults to guide children's behavior so it is acceptable, these behaviors are common ways of demonstrating curiosity and do not typically indicate unhealthy sexuality development (Schuhrke 2000).

Understanding how very young children develop socially and emotionally

Erik Erikson's (1963) theory provides information about social and emotional development across the life span. In his work Erikson theorized

that, during the first year of life, resolving the issue of trust is the most important issue, and its resolution allows healthy personality development (Erikson 1963). Infants who learn to trust the adults who care for them during this developmental period are on a path to positive growth. Trust is taught by meeting the needs of infants in a responsive way. When needs are met, infants begin the developmental course to a sense of self-worth. One can extract from earlier discussions of Greenspan's (1990) developmental view that trust is very important to later healthy sexuality development.

Erikson's second stage of social and emotional development involves toddlers' learning to trust themselves, or the establishment of autonomy (Erikson 1963). To successfully reach this developmental milestone, toddlers need adults who encourage them to do things for themselves and provide necessary support to help the toddler with the accomplishment. Additionally, during this stage, toddlers need adults who will set reasonable and fairly consistent limits on behavior. When adults provide a good balance between encouragement and limit setting, toddlers gain in their ability to do things for themselves, which in turn, leads to a heightened sense of self-esteem. By age 3, children who feel a sense

Healthy Sexuality Development

of self-worth are more capable of respecting others and taking responsibility.

Understanding how children with developmental disabilities develop healthy sexuality

The information in this chapter assumes typical development in children. This section, excerpted from an article that appeared in *The SIECUS Report*, provides facts about healthy sexuality development in infants and toddlers with disabilities:

Children with developmental disabilities may learn at slower rates than their nondisabled peers, but their physical maturation typically occurs at the normal stages of development. The sexual maturation of children with disabilities does, however, have some noted differences. As result, their parents need to understand what to expect at different stages of psychosexual development, from infancy onward, in order to understand be appropriateness of their children's sexual behaviors and expression.

Infants possess the physiology for arousal and orgasm and the capacity for a variety of sexual behaviors beginning at or before birth. During infancy, the experience of sucking and being cradled is of critical importance to the child's sexual development. When infants have a developmental disability, this experience may be delayed or restricted due to their medical needs. When infants have a disability that interferes with their capacity to give appropriate cues to their parents, parental bonding and subsequent attachment are often inhibited. Regardless of their level of bonding and stimulation, infants with developmental disabilities demonstrate delays in distinguishing body feelings from other feelings, in differentiating among parts of the body, and in engaging in distinctive genital sexual play. As children with developmental disabilities move from infancy to the toddler and preschool years, a myriad of issues emerge concerning psychosexual development. Toilet training often occurs at a late age and over longer period of time, thus causing delays in their developing self-control and a sense of self.

The sense of self of children with developmental disabilities is further delayed as a result of an elongated period of dependency on parents or caregivers for personal care and hygiene. This often leads to their inability to differentiate between the sexual and nonsexual parts of their bodies. As a result, children with developmental disabilities may not firmly understand body ownership since they are not allowed to own even the nonsexual parts of their bodies.

Such lack of body ownership may result in children with developmental disabilities being confused about their sexual selves. This developmental lag in distinguishing the self as separate from parent/caregiver is reflected in the delayed rate at which children develop perceptions of themselves as either boys or girls. At later developmental stages, children with developmental disabilities are able to self-identify as male or female and to develop sex-role identity. (Ballan 2001, 15–16)

Guidelines

The guidelines that are presented in this section must be considered in light of the critical role that important adults play in the earliest development of healthy sexuality. These guidelines are broad in nature and hold true for parents, other family members, and caregivers:

Be understanding of children's curiosity about their bodies and other children's bodies. It is as natural as their curiosity about other common items in their environment (Honig 2000).

Demonstrate acceptance of all bodies and bodily functions. Explain that elimination is natural and that everyone does it.

Provide appropriate care for children. This includes healthy nutrition, supervision for safety, good hygiene, medical attention for wellness and illness, appropriate demonstrations of affection, positive attitudes, and modeling of appropriate ways to express feelings.

Teach that all people are worthy of respect. When children call attention to differences such as gender, abilities, race, and so forth, acknowledge the difference in a positive way.

Support children in their building of friendships by modeling social interaction. Casual, caring, and relaxed communication and settings help children and adults build relationships.

Provide a variety of active and quiet play choices for all children. Encourage varied and multiple interests at play.

Attend to your own attitudes about sex. Learn to accept your body (Honig 2000).

Be aware of your reactions to children's behaviors and comments about sex. Practice calm reactions (Honig 2000).

Planning for healthy sexuality development for infants and toddlers

Obviously, caregivers and teachers should be prepared to carry out each of the general guidelines listed above. In addition, they should understand long-term influences they will have on children's development. In particular, they should model good hygiene and appropriate way to express feelings. Their support of children's friendships and appropriate expressions of affection is fundamentally important. They must also be prepared to communicate with families about sensitive issues related to sexuality.

As they organize their classrooms and child care settings, teachers and caregivers need to consider how the setting and activities could support the development of the whole child (for example, creating active and quiet areas and providing a variety of toys, materials, books, puzzles). The settings can convey a respect for differences through displays of pictures showing various family structures, ethnic groups, differently abled people, as well as males and females in a variety of roles, especially roles showing females in positions of leadership.

Working with families

Some family members are likely to be uncomfortable initiating a discussion about any topic relating to healthy sexuality in very young children. In many cases, the early childhood teacher, caregiver, or administrator will likely need to provide information to families in appropriate formats and at the right time. Some of this information can be placed in a newsletter, parent or family handbook, flyer, or brochure. Other information might better be shared in a workshop or discussion group format. Some families will benefit from other publications and media that you can identify and make available.

Topics that will be particularly relevant include the following:

• **Diapering and toilet learning.** Especially consider preparing written information on these subjects.

• **Children's curiosity, especially about genitals and about self-touching of genitals.** Include guidelines stating that, at this age, the touching of children's genitals by anyone other than the child him- or herself should be done only for hygienic or medical purposes.

• **Differences between children's sexuality development and adult views of sexuality.** Characteristics of children's sexuality include curiosity, playfulness and openness; adult sexuality is based on knowledge and must be concerned with consequences of behavior and privacy (Rothbaum, Grauer, & Rubin 1997).

• **Ways for parents and other family members to fulfill their most important role as sexuality educators to their family's own young children.** Recommended sources for families are found in the Resources section.

• **Antibias approaches that families and staff can use to provide an inclusive setting that respects and accepts various cultural differences and family structures.** The *Anti-Bias Curriculum* (Derman-Sparks & the A.B.C. Task Force 1989) is an important tool.

Behaviors and attitudes to avoid

All adults should avoid expressing or modeling the following behaviors or attitudes, especially to young children:

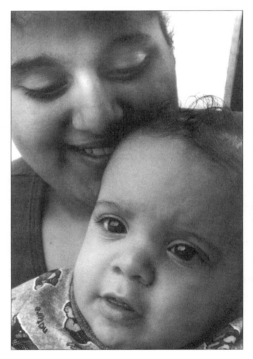

• Implying or communicating that some body parts are bad or shameful

• Conveying that the child is bad or naughty because of an action or word

• Communicating to families that their children are bad or abnormal because of something the children say or do

• Assigning to children's interest in sexuality interpretations that are related to adult sexuality

• Demonstrating biases toward people

Healthy Sexuality Development

＊　　＊　　＊

Sexuality, even as early as infancy and toddler-
hood, is a normal part of being human. No
amount of ignoring or denying reality will change
that fact. Teachers and parents can support or
inhibit young children's healthy sexuality development through their attitudes, interactions, and
other behaviors.

Adults who work with young children have a
responsibility to optimize children's well-being. By
attending to their own uneasiness about sex, early
childhood professionals can better understand and
support healthy sexuality development in young
children. Because adult attitudes and behaviors
influence all aspects of children's development tre-
mendously and because more young children than
ever are spending greater amounts of time in early
childhood education programs, early childhood
educators are wise to increase their understanding
and skills related to healthy sexuality development.

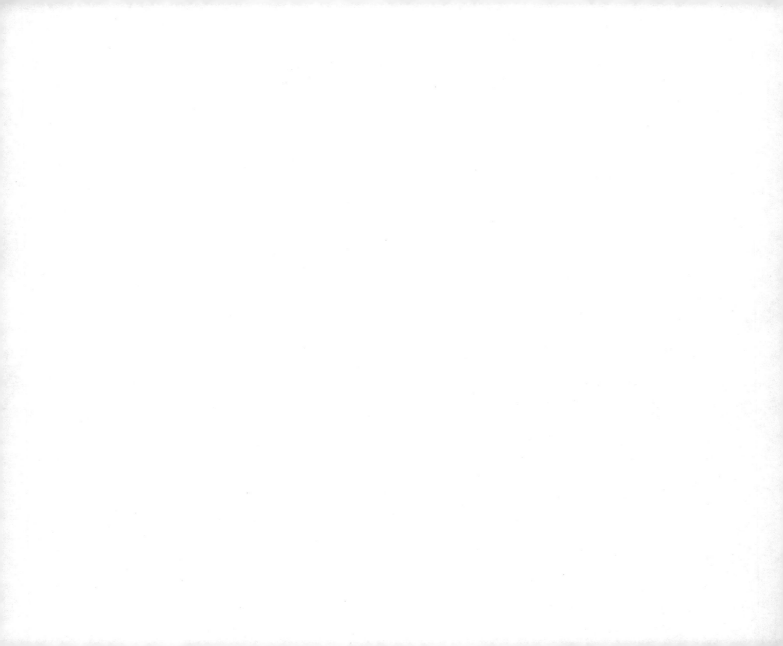

3

Preschoolers

In each of the following scenarios and in the thousands that occur each day, teachers must decide how they will react. Their decisions play a critical role in the sexuality development of the children in their care.

Eve and Josh are playing in the dramatic play area. Both children have recently had births in their families, and both children were at the hospital during the delivery of their new siblings. The teacher observes Josh and Eve acting out the birth process by pretending that a baby doll is moving down their bodies and coming out between their legs. This activity is done with sound and excited motions.

Benjamin and his preschool teacher are sitting together on the bench at recess. They are talking about Benjamin's friends and play preferences. The teacher is helping him make a choice about play partners. Benjamin says to the teacher that he does not like to play with the boys and that he most likes to play with Nicole and Shana. The teacher asks him what kinds of things he likes to do. He says that he likes to swing, play in the sandbox, and sit on the climber.

Elaine tells her mom that she wants to wear only pants and shirts and does not want to wear dresses. Her mom asks to talk with the classroom teacher about her daughter's preference and expresses concern about what it means. During the conference with the teacher, Elaine's mom also tells the teacher that Elaine prefers to play only with boys and seeks out the most active games to play—play that mom classifies as "boy games"—and finally labels Elaine as a "tomboy."

Each of these scenes requires the teacher to choose what action to take. One choice is to make an accepting, nonintrusive response that allows children to act out or express their thoughts and feelings without adult involvement. A second course of action is for the teacher to support or extend the play or dialogue by asking questions, suggesting actions, or giving options. A third choice for the teacher is to actively redirect, stop, or take control of the situation, removing any choice from the children. A box showing possible actions is found below. In the following sections of this chapter, information is provided to assist classroom teachers in making decisions and taking actions that support young children's healthy sexuality development in preschool settings.

Developmental understandings

Young children's play preferences, social interactions, and physical actions are not dependable predictors of sexual activity or sexual orientation in adolescence or adulthood. However, "sexuality is central to being human" (SIECUS Early Childhood Task Force 1998, 45). Thus, at all ages, sexuality is a primary characteristic of human beings, even though we observe essential differences between children's sexuality and adults' sexuality. Adults are knowing and aware of consequences whereas children are curious and playful; adults are self-conscious and desire privacy and children are spontaneous and open; adults are

Choices for Action with Respect to

Responding to child behaviors with minimal guidance (redirection or prohibition)	Contacting family about child behavior	Designing policies, staff training events; collecting resources and information about sexuality development	Involving other professionals, for example, pediatricians, psychologists, counselors, social workers, child development and human sexuality specialists

motivated by eroticism whereas children are superficial in their sensuality (their sensuality is not motivated by sexual desire and is often an imitation of observed adult behavior) (Rothbaum, Grauer, & Rubin 1997). Best practice in early childhood education holds that parents and teachers who are accepting of children's constructive play preferences and interests support children's developing sense of self and help to build their self-esteem.

By encouraging young children to make choices about clothing, friendships, and activities, we are promoting independence, social skills, and greater understanding of life experiences. With this type of encouragement from families and caregivers, children feel safe and secure in their learning environments. Physical and psychological safety

are necessary for supporting children's healthy development in all areas, including sexuality.

An audiotape produced by the Association for Supervision and Curriculum Development (ASCD), titled *Sexual Orientation Issues in the Curriculum,* states a mission of schools: "Schools should be safe, protected, comfortable environments with an emphasis on diversity and meeting the needs of all students" (Pietrzak et al. 2000). This mission suggests that young children's behaviors, actions, and words should be understood in a context that is based on age characteristics, individual personality and temperament, family, and community. This contextual understanding is also influenced by the children's physical, cognitive, and social development. The information outlined in "Developmental

Sexuality Development in Programs for Young Children

Involving families in the planning, decision making, and providing of resources	Planning developmentally appropriate curriculum that includes healthy sexuality content and a plan for family involvement	Planning schoolwide programs about typical development, including sexuality

Physical development

- Uses correct names for parts of the body
- Deals with some toilet training challenges (either standing or sitting)
- Experiences touching of genitalia for pleasure (including masturbation)
- Appreciates various sensory experiences
- Experiences rapid growth and physical change
- Practices independence and self-care, including routines to stay healthy and well (toileting, handwashing, and so on)

Cognitive development

- Understands that boys and girls have similarities and differences in bodies
- Notices physical differences between girls and boys
- Recognizes that bodies come in many sizes and shapes
- Is curious about her or his own body functions and sex differences

- Shows interest in reproduction, birth, how adults become parents
- Continues to learn about interpersonal relationships, expressions of affection
- Understands that some adults are married and some are single
- Knows proper terms for body parts as well as processes and uses these terms appropriately

Social development

- Realizes that families care for children
- Is aware that families come in various forms
- Knows that children may have one family or more than one family with whom they reside
- Recognizes and accepts that people have different abilities, interests, talents, skills
- Increases ability to establish friendships
- Often engages in same-gender play activities by about 3 1/2 years (Maccoby 1998)
- Feels free to engage in play based on his or her own interests

Sexuality for the Preschool Child

- Often interacts with boys and girls in different ways
- Demonstrates individual personality characteristics
- Acts in masculine or feminine ways, according to his or her own gender and expectations of families and cultures
- Can attend to issues of diversity and equity, including fairness, social justice, cooperation

Emotional development

- Begins to develop understanding of self, including gender identity, (which continues to develop throughout the life span)
- Develops positive self-esteem
- Expresses positive feelings about bodies
- Accepts and expresses love, care, and affection
- Can express feelings in appropriate ways
- Shows a developing sense of empathy when opportunities exist

Expectations Related to Healthy Sexuality for the Preschool Child" reviews milestones for each developmental process as it relates to healthy sexuality development in children ages 3 to 5 years.

Many preschool children are in child care and other out-of-home settings for much of their day. It is likely then that caregivers, teachers, and administrators will have occurrences of sexuality-related language, behavior, or questions and will have more responsibility for sexuality education than in the past. Examples of this responsibility include responding to the questions of young children and their families as well as establishing guidelines for appropriate behaviors. The increase in numbers of children in early childhood education settings, these children's greater diversity in life experiences, and varying family values are all factors creating a need for early childhood professionals to demonstrate sensitivity and tolerance when considering matters related to healthy sexuality.

Educational responsibilities include understanding preschool development with respect to sexuality and planning a variety of experiences and activities that promote healthy attitudes and behaviors. The suggestions listed below are included to help teachers prepare for planned activities and to provide a broader understanding of development. General guidelines for responding to children's behavior or questions relating to sexuality include the following:

• When interacting with children, consistently use correct terms such as *penis, vulva, egg, sperm, urination, defecation,* but do not require children to use these terms themselves in all situations. Acknowledge and talk about the various words that children sometimes use for these terms.

• Use a calm voice when discussing sexuality, not one that is hysterical, judgmental, or out of control.

• Be child centered and age appropriate. Avoid using an adult frame of reference with respect to sexuality or giving adult meaning to children's actions or words. Try to understand the child's point of view, experiences, and concerns.

Understanding the sexuality development of preschoolers with developmental disabilities

The information in this chapter is applicable to working with typically developing preschool children. This section, excerpted from an article that appeared in *The SIECUS Report,* provides information for understanding the needs that preschoolers with developmental disabilities may have with respect to sexuality development.

Upon reaching preschool age, children with developmental disabilities exhibit a heightened level of curiosity about others and about sexual differences between males and females. Their curiosity is, however, less intense than their nondisabled peers. Children with developmental disabilities may not be allowed to resolve their curiosity due to prolonged supervision. At this stage of psychosexual development, they often experience problems differentiating between private and public places and actions and therefore may engage in publicly unacceptable sexual behaviors. Children with developmental disabilities are often unaware of what sexual behaviors are appropriate due to limited social interactions and lack opportunities to observe or model behaviors of their nondisabled peers. (Ballan 2001, 16)

Valuing preschool children's social play

In high-quality preschool programs, children are provided with a great deal of time to engage in play. Play, as defined by Rubin, Fein, and Vandenberg (1983), is children's activity that is internally motivated, free of external rules, carried out as if it were real, focused on the process (not the product), as well as chosen and directed by the players. A large body of observational research has documented that, during the preschool years, children frequently prefer same-sex play partners and choose activities that are traditionally geared to either boys or girls (Maccoby 1998). Research (Maccoby 1998) shows what many preschool teachers observe on a regular basis in their classrooms:

• By the age of 3 years, children spend most of their time with same-sex peers.

• By the age of 4 years, both boys and girls demonstrate a clear preference for same-sex playmates.

• By 5 years of age, boys show a stronger preference for same-sex playmates.

Children not only show clear gender preferences in their playmates but also exhibit differences in styles of play (see "Typical Play Styles").

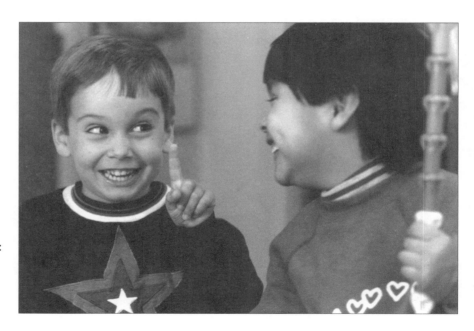

Gender Differences in Play

The consistent differences found in the play of girls and boys should not lead to stereotypes such as "boys don't like to play house" or "girls don't like physical play." Children of either gender may vary substantially in their individual preferences. At the same time, researchers regularly observe gender differences in children's style of play (Maccoby 1998). Teachers' awareness of such differences helps to ensure that they support and encourage the full range of play enjoyed by both girls and boys and respect individual differences.

Typical Play Styles

Girls	*Boys*
Play in groups of two or three	Play in large groups
Prefer inside play	Prefer outside play
Are more cooperative	Are rougher, more physical
Show concern for others in distress	Are more competitive
In conflict, use social alienation	By 3 years, use more direct aggression
Often play close to adults	Avoid proximity to adults

Frequent Play Themes

Family	Heroic characters
School	Danger
Nurturance	Righteous combat
Adornment	Action

Further, Maccoby (1998) notes differences in play themes for girls and boys as they engage in pretense (see "Typical Play Themes").

For several decades now, preschool teachers have been perplexed about how to deal with child-selected gender segregation in the classroom. In the 1970s, many teachers attempted to assign boys to play areas that typically attract girls and to assign girls to play areas that typically attract boys. The results were disturbing to some observers when boys treated dolls like airplanes and girls turned the climbing apparatuses into family huts. Although well intended, this approach does not effectively promote sexuality development in a holistic, integrated way. To best serve the needs of all children, teachers should

• provide an array choices compatible with the interests and styles of all children's play;

• encourage play styles and themes of both girls and boys in all areas of the indoor and outdoor environment;

• use direct and indirect guidance strategies to support individual choices and group preferences; and,

• elicit inclusive attitudes and behaviors through the use of an antibias approach in the classroom.

Teachers need to understand both the nature of children's play and the nature of gender roles with preschool children. Although many children exhibit preferences that are traditional for their gender, individual differences must be accommodated in preschool settings. "Focus on children first, issues second" (Dispenza 1999, 20) is a useful guideline for teachers' decision making. Assigning children to play areas based on gender or expecting any particular boy to prefer themes of action over nurturance and any particular girl to prefer themes of adornment over superheroes does not encourage children to make their own choices. Teachers can support individual differences in play preferences and styles through their attitudes as well as through the curriculum and instructional strategies. This support will lead children to a positive sense of self and toward acceptance of differences.

Preschool children are notoriously curious. This curiosity is often demonstrated in their pretend play. Typically, children play out their interests. As the first scenario in this chapter demonstrates, both boys and girls may pretend to give birth. Sometimes, preschool children initiate cooperative play that is sexual in nature. Depending on children's life experiences, teachers may observe children showing their genitals to others or even touching another child's genitalia. Often, this commonplace behavior occurs between children of the opposite sex because children are interested in and curious about differences.

Guidelines

Greenspan's (1990) developmental sequence of pleasure and sexuality emphasizes the strong interest that preschool children have in their own bodies. These early feelings that children have about their bodies are related to both healthy sexuality development and character development. Children's increasing ability to appreciate reality allows them to internalize and represent early attitudes about their bodies in more complex ways. Adults who reject children or punish behavior related to children's interest in their bodies may negatively influence children's healthy sexuality development. When teachers have needed to provide guidance to children with respect to this behavior, many have found that an effective strategy is to calmly and matter-of-factly redirect children to another activity. Attentive supervision during play time is necessary not only for keeping children safe but also for extending play in meaningful and supportive ways.

Teachers of young children often are concerned about differentiating between typical behaviors related to sex play for young children and those behaviors that are more indicative of abuse.

Children who have been sexually abused may demonstrate more intrusive kinds of behavior such as forced penetration or oral-genital contact with other children (Wardle 1998). This kind of behavior is not based on a child's natural curiosity and requires teachers to report the possibility of child abuse according to their state policy.

The following list provides helpful guidelines teachers can follow to ensure children's well-being.

Take several steps if a child is touching his or her genitals in public. Make sure the child is aware of the behavior, acknowledge that it feels good but is to be done in private, and help the child identify "public" and "private" settings (SIECUS Early Childhood Task Force 1998).

Act promptly to stop certain behaviors. Attend to any child-to-child behavior that is inappropriate, intrusive, or painful; any self-inflicted painful sexual activity; and any oral-genital contact or forced penetration with an object or a finger (Wardle 1998). Follow through with appropriate reporting procedures.

Encourage children to speak up. Let them know they can and should tell a friend, an older child, a teacher, or a parent if they do not like what someone is doing to them or to their body.

Make sure children are aware that each person can decide whether he or she wants to be hugged or touched (in appropriately affectionate ways). Repeat the phrase, "Your body belongs to you," frequently when interacting with children in different situations.

Planning experiences and activities for healthy sexuality development

Teachers should make children aware of the variety that occurs among family structures and practices as well as in body types. Activities or communications might include the following:

• Group times that feature stories about a variety of families

• Group times to which pregnant women and mothers who have recently given birth are invited

• Opportunities to share photos of babies and families

• Displays (that are changed frequently) in each of the centers around the room, which show a variety of body types

In addition, teachers should explain ways to stay healthy and have children practice hygienic procedures such as handwashing, wiping after toileting, nose blowing, and so forth, in authentic situations. In these situations, teachers would, for example, explain that urination and defecation are normal ways that a body works and would teach girls to wipe with toilet tissue from front to back after urinating and to use a separate piece of toilet tissue to wipe buttocks from front to back. Teachers should assist in cleaning up toileting accidents in a noncritical way, avoiding reprimands, shame-provoking remarks, and statements indicating frustration. In these situations, teachers might tell the child that "these things happen" or say, "We'll just clean it up, get some different clothes, and then you can go back and play."

Working with families

Effective early childhood educators are aware that forming partnerships with families of the children they teach is important. Substantial evidence points to the fact that families are the primary force in children's development (Couchenour & Chrisman 2000a). Experts in sexuality education believe strongly that parents are children's most important sex educators (SIECUS 1998). Preschool teachers and administrators can effectively work with families to support children's healthy sexuality development by doing the following:

• Help parents to understand children's natural curiosity about their bodies and about how they were conceived and born.

• Provide information proactively—before possible situations arise that may be sensitive or cause embarrassment to parents.

• Make print and electronic resources available for families.

• Include a section in the parent handbook about teaching strategies and school policy with respect to children's healthy sexuality development.

• Form a committee or task force of diverse family and community members to ensure that concerns of all families are met in ways that best support children. (See "Staff Development 6," p. 74, for specific ideas for situations in which parents and caregivers differ sharply in their perspectives and negotiation is needed.)

When working with lesbian, gay, bisexual, and transgender families, it is important to maintain an attitude of openness and respect, to provide policies that support all families, and to seek professional training as needed to increase understanding that leads to inclusive practices. In a study to identify the best practices in child care for lesbian, gay, bisexual, and transgender families, the Lesbian and Gay Child Care Task Force (Dispenza 1999) collected information about the practices in child care settings that resulted in positive actions or events for these families. Some of the emergent practices that the families found to be positive included the following:

• Creating a welcoming environment for all families

• Appreciating diversity and differences

• Fostering a sensitive staff that responds to all families

• Updating policies, handbooks, and newsletters so they reflect openness to all family configurations

• Knowing that exclusion hurts children

• Accepting families unconditionally

• Honoring with positive attitudes the specific requests of family members

• Respecting the rights of others

• Being willing to change to increase inclusivity

• Taking conscientious steps to diminish fear and misunderstanding about homosexuality

• Showing a willingness to overcome homophobia (Dispenza 1999)

Behaviors and attitudes to avoid

The previous chapter describes behaviors for adults to avoid in interacting with infants and toddlers; similar cautions apply with preschoolers. Adults should never imply to children that they are bad or naughty because of their natural curiosity about their own bodies, or topics such as pregnancy and birth. When interpreting children's words or actions, teachers must remember that children do not possess adult knowledge or motivations. Moreover, even as preschoolers become more aware of gender differences, adults should be careful not limit children's play to traditional gender-specific roles.

❋　　❋　　❋

Understanding typical and age-appropriate sexuality characteristics of preschool children can help teachers, caregivers, administrators, and families to plan programs, respond to questions, and interact knowledgeably. When sexuality is viewed as part and parcel of human development, it loses its mystique and takes its rightful place as an integral part of each child's development.

4

Primary-Age Children

The following scenarios are typical situations when working with primary-age children.

During recess on the playground, girls and boys in first grade have been playing in gender-segregated groups. The teacher notices that suddenly boys and girls begin to interact with one another in games of chase.

Throughout the week, behaviors get a little more verbally and physically aggressive each day. The play continues to be somewhat segregated in that boys are the chasers and girls are being chased.

At dinner one evening, 7-year-old Celeste is eating with her parents and 5-year-old brother, Caleb, when she puts down her fork and asks, "Dad, what is sex?" After several moments of silence, Paul, Celeste's dad, says, "Let's finish dinner so we can go outside and play some catch before it gets dark." Later that evening, Paul and Arlene, Celeste's mom, wonder what is going on at school that has led to their daughter's question about sex. They call Celeste's teacher the next day to get some answers.

Jennifer is a first-year teacher of a third-grade class that includes Reba. Reba's mother, Anya, calls Jennifer at home one evening to tell her that, according to Reba, Chad has been smacking Reba and several other girls on their "bottoms" and now has begun to pat their chests while commenting on "girl boobs." Jennifer listened politely to Anya's concerns and then began to search for information about appropriate ways to intervene in this situation at school. She did not feel comfortable asking anyone for advice or information about children and sex.

When such situations occur, teachers who understand child development—and specifically development of sexuality—will be prepared and take advantage of the teaching opportunities these events offer. For other teachers, these events present a challenge, but also the opportunity for learning and for personal and professional growth.

Children in primary grades often demonstrate strong preferences for playing with children of their own gender. Reasons for this behavior are not completely known; however, as noted in Chapter 3, evidence (Maccoby 1998) points to the notions that play themes and play styles differ by gender beginning at the age of 3. Girls often engage in themes related to family, school, or adornment whereas boys engage in themes involving action, danger, and heroism. Girls' play styles typically show greater cooperation, smaller groups, and closer proximity to teachers or other adults; boys play in larger groups, are more competitive, and avoid proximity to adults (Maccoby 1998). By the primary years, many children likely have become accustomed to gender-specific play themes and play styles and may have difficulty negotiating how to play together in mixed-gender groups.

Further, Maccoby (1998) reports that, in middle childhood (ages 6–10 years), boys increase their use of inappropriate or "dirty" language, often making homophobic comments, talking about girls' bodies, and uttering explicit sexual terms. At this age, boys also ridicule girls and typically label certain behaviors as being feminine. Although some girls engage in what is incorrectly referred to as "tomboy" activi-

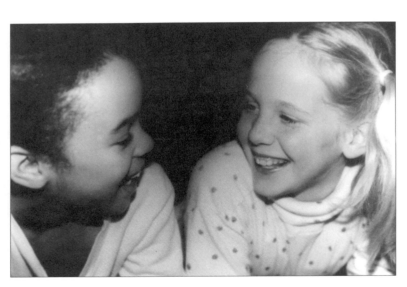

ties and seem to be comfortable around boys, girls more commonly are wary of boys and avoid them. Although the two sexes tend to remain separate during this period, they seem to be very aware of each other, and both groups may tease others about having boyfriends or girlfriends, being in love, and getting married. Interestingly, at this point in their development, this teasing generally assumes only heterosexual relationships.

Developmental understandings

Children between the ages of 6 and 8 years were believed by Freud (1917) to be in a stage of latency, meaning that children are not actively concerned with issues of sexuality. Although it may be true that sexuality is not as significant during this period as it is likely to become during puberty, contemporary developmental views of children's healthy sexuality do not identify a period that can be accurately called latency. Ryan's (2000) review of the literature notes that naturalistic research from more "primitive" cultures documents substantial sexual interest prior to puberty. Today, child development specialists are asking whether the concept of latency is indeed a developmental phenomenon or whether children simply have been led to react to adult silence and secrecy about sexuality in behaviors that support the latency concept.

Greenspan notes that "sexual issues during latency are not so latent" (1990, 51). Children in the primary grades continue to be very interested in sexual differences between girls and boys and may be very curious, often exhibiting what is termed a "precocious adolescent preoccupation" with using prohibited language (which causes giggling) and looking at pictures of men or women who are wearing little or no clothing. When adults are understanding and supportive in their interactions—even in their corrections—with children, healthy sexuality can flourish. However, when adults have extreme discomfort with children's interests during this period or when they become either aloof or overinvolved in the children's striving for pleasure, their behavior may interfere with the children's healthy sexuality development. To optimize this sexuality development, adults must understand all aspects of children's development that relate to healthy, age-appropriate sexuality.

Gender differences are often so established and ingrained in children by the time they enter primary grades that both girls and boys may have difficulty getting beyond the stereotypes unless caring adults intervene and provide information. The preference for same-sex playmates and friendships continues throughout this period; these preferences are very strong and they frequently lead to gender segregation at school. Very likely, many boys and girls have such disparate school experiences that they may seem to have grown up in two different cultures (Maccoby 1998).

Cognitively, children of this age are entering Piaget's ([1936] 1952) concrete operational stage. Many children progress from preoperational thinking to concrete operational thinking near the end of first grade. One of the new characteristics that emerges during this period is the ability to decenter, that is, to consider more than one object, event, or idea at a time. With this emerging ability, children's egocentric thinking decreases. Consequently, children can understand that, even though some adults may disagree about gender expectations, it is all right for some girls to prefer highly active play and for some boys to prefer quiet, calm play. The ability to decenter also permits the child to realize that gender alone does not provide all the information about an individual.

At this time, too, children begin to have a firmer grasp of rules. When this ability is new, children are sometimes very rigid with rules, so the notion that all activities are appropriate for both girls and boys may need to be guided and supported by teachers and parents. For example, 5-year-old Christopher was showing his Aunt Dee his new toy, a big yellow truck that, at the push of a button, dumped its contents. Aunt Dee said, "I like that truck. I want one just like it." Christopher's response was, "Aunt Dee, I'd share my truck with you, but it's only for boys." Through discussions, stories, and real-life experiences, adults can help children to understand that toys can be selected by either boys or girls, depending on their interests.

The development of empathy, the ability to consider how another person might be feeling, is also a part of this cognitive transformation. When children have been encouraged previously by adults to attend to feelings of others, they typically have the ability in the primary grades to make judgments and to respond in appropriate ways to the distress of another (Santrock 2001). Thus, adults may point out to children at this age how their behavior might positively or negatively affect another person. At earlier stages of development, this approach is often not as beneficial.

At this age, children also become more capable of understanding causal connections. One result is that children can better grasp the concept of the reproductive process. Information about sexual intercourse and the possible result of sperm and ovum uniting might begin to make some sense. This understanding differs from the understanding that Vivian Paley (1981) writes about in *Wally's Stories*. In Paley's book, one of the kindergarten children reported that her aunt was going to have a baby. When asked how the baby got inside her aunt, she replied, "She wished for it." Additionally, she noted that it was okay for her aunt to wish for the baby because she was "past high school." In contrast, children who are in the concrete operational stage (beginning at about age 7) can begin to understand reproduction more accurately in terms of cause and effect—the

uniting of sperm and egg as an early step to having a baby.

"Developmental Expectations Related to Healthy Sexuality for Children Ages 6 through 8 Years" on pages 56–58 summarizes information from a variety of resources, including materials from SIECUS.

Understanding sexuality development of primary-age children with developmental disabilities

Information in this chapter is especially relevant for typically developing children. Ballan provides facts with respect to sexuality development of primary-age children with developmental disabilities:

As a result of the media and their peers, children with developmental disabilities confront the school years with an increased awareness of their sexuality. However, during this time, their social activities remain closely supervised, and normal sexual expressions of behavior are often discouraged. They tend not to ask questions about sexuality, but when they do they often articulate the questions poorly due to an undeveloped sexual vocabulary. At this

Developmental Expectations Related to Healthy Sexuality

Physical development

• Grows taller and heavier (girls lag but catch up by the end of third grade [Trawick-Smith 1997])
• Slims down if body is still roundish
• May masturbate; knows it feels good and understands privacy issues
• May become more modest about his or her body, depending on the home environment
• Continues to practice good hygienic care
• Experiences changes in body with age

Cognitive development

• Focuses on how peers' bodies and appearances differ
• Shows curiosity about his or her own body
• Knows the names and functions for all body parts
• Learns that good health habits can improve the way he or she looks and feels
• Understands that HIV is usually acquired during adult sexual behavior or use of shared injected drugs and that it is not contagious through ordinary contact with someone who has AIDS
• Realizes that bodies of boys and girls are more alike than different
• Recognizes that boys and girls have different genitals, reproductive organs, genes
• Can specify that males have a penis, scrotum, and testicles and that females have a vulva, clitoris, vagina, uterus, and ovaries
• Knows that reproduction requires both sperm and ovum
• Understands that reproductive organs in men and women enable them to have a child
• Is aware that, when a woman is pregnant, the fetus grows inside her uterus
• Knows that babies are born from a woman's body through an opening called the vagina
• Can explain that sexual intercourse occurs when a man and woman place the penis inside the vagina
• Knows that women have breasts that can provide milk for a baby

for a Child Ages 6 through 8 Years

• Understands that everyone is born a boy or girl and that boys grow up to be men and girls grow up to be women

• Is aware that most people are "heterosexual, which means they will be attracted to and fall in love with someone of the other gender" and that some people are "homosexual, which means they will be attracted to and fall in love with someone of the same gender" (SIECUS National Guidelines Task Force 1996, 15)

• Knows that not everything on television, in movies or books, or on the Internet is true

• Is aware that advertisements are trying to sell products and that they often make people and things look better than they are in reality

Social development

• Is aware that a person expresses love and affection in different ways depending on his or her relationship with the other person (i.e., friend, parent, sibling)

• Is aware that adults often kiss, hug, and touch to show caring for one another

• Considers bodies of both girls and boys to be equally admirable

• Knows that families have rules about helping one another

• Recognizes that families are not all alike, for example, families have different numbers of adults and children in them and family members may not all live in the same place

• Knows that in families adults care for children

• Knows that raising children is an adult responsibility

• Knows that sexual intercourse is for adults, not children

• Recognizes that people have many kinds of relationships involving families, friends, dating, falling in love, marriage

• Recognizes that many couples marry to share their lifetime commitment to each other and that some people choose lifetime commitments but do not marry

• Is aware that sometimes people who marry get divorced

Developmental Expectations Related to Healthy Sexuality for Children Ages 6 through 8 Years (cont'd)

Social development (cont'd)

• Recognizes that resolving conflicts keeps relationships healthy

• Understands that males and females can do almost all of the same jobs and housekeeping tasks

• Knows that both mothers and fathers are important as parents

• Understands that all people should be treated fairly

• Recognizes differences in people and through ongoing discussions with adults increasingly understands and values others

• Is aware that some television programs, movies, books, and Internet sites are not appropriate for children

Emotional development

• Is aware that all families hold strong beliefs or values but that families do not all have the same values

• Is aware that religions often teach values but that not all religions teach the same values

• Knows that choices have consequences

• Trusts that most adults can help children to make good choices

• Knows that telling a trusted adult about his or her feelings and needs is important

• Knows that if his or her parent cannot help, he or she can ask a teacher, religious leader, guidance counselor, a friend's parent, or another trusted adult

• Knows that children and adults have rights

• Knows that everyone has the right to tell others not to touch their bodies when they do not want to be touched stage of their sexual maturation, children with developmental disabilities frequently masturbate. Parents of these children have reported that their children between the ages of six and ten "frequently" touch their genitals. Children with developmental disabilities are often overcorrected for masturbating, and later may experience guilt and uneasiness. (2001,16)

Guidelines

The following general guidelines provide adults with a productive and healthy approach to fostering healthy sexuality development in primary-age children. Each of the guidelines is discussed in more depth in the sections that follow:

Take into account children's cognitive abilities. Primary-age children have the emerging ability to understand the feelings of others and to realize the importance of taking responsibility for their own actions. Although individual differences in children's abilities must be considered, adults can provide support to help children build their strengths in these areas. Children at this age can learn to recognize feelings of others and then to imagine how others might feel in various situations. Children can then identify ways that they might interact with others to create a positive outcome. Adults can support children's efforts by planning a curriculum around the themes of caring or responsibility and by behavioral interventions in the form of reminders or small group discussions.

In addition, creating rules or expectations for children at home and at school is useful. Often, classroom rules suggest minimal expectations for behavior. When adults hold and communicate higher expectations for children, many times they quickly rise to the occasion. These expectations might be communicated to children as follows:

• Consider how your words or actions might make someone else feel.

• Think before acting.

• Remember that your choices have consequences.

• Choose a respectful solution.

• Care for others.

Model and expect positive, appropriate interactions with others. One of the best reasons to use positive guidance or discipline approaches with primary-age children is that doing it allows adults to model respectful interaction with others. In contrast, when adults yell or use corporal punishment, children are likely to imitate those actions with others. Remind children to consider the feelings of others by putting themselves in "the other person's shoes." Using stories to support empathic responses might be helpful. Some books that might be especially effective include the following:

Asha's Mums by R. Elwin and M. Paulse

History of Women for Children by V. S. Epstein

How Would You Feel If Your Dad Was Gay?
   by A. Heron and M. Maran

Just Us Women by J. Caines

Oliver Button Is a Sissy by T. dePaola

Snow Woman by D. McKee

The Sneetches by Dr. Seuss

William's Doll by C. Zolotow

Stop aggression and bullying on the spot.
Ignoring aggressive behavior or bullying is equiva-lent to condoning the hurtful actions by being silent. Children need parents, teachers, and other important adults in their lives to remind them to stop when they are hurting others. Recent events of violence in schools have taught us that the old adage "Sticks and stones may break my bones, but words will never hurt me" has no ring of truth to it. Words can hurt. Children must be taught this fact by the adults who care for them.

Note children's preferences for same-gender groups. The fact that young children often prefer to work and play in same-gender groups has been widely documented (Maccoby 1998). This phenomenon can create so much concern that parents or teachers often report as troublesome the boy who prefers playing with girls or the girl who prefers playing with boys. This preference that is typical of primary-age children can pose a bit of a dilemma for adults. We know that, to increase one's understanding of others, getting firsthand experience with those others is helpful. Thus, a common approach has been for teachers to pair a child with one of the opposite gender or to require groups to be made up of both boys and girls. Many teachers have found that this forced ap-

Healthy Sexuality Development

proach is actually unproductively confining and often backfires in some way. Teachers may find that a more successful way to integrate their classrooms by gender is to provide access to a variety of topics and teaching or learning methods, which leads to more authentic gender integration. For example, when children are choosing project themes, a teacher might consider providing choices that provide for a rich variety of interests and abilities.

Do not ignore the "sex talk." When children are calling attention to body parts or sexual acts in a way that intimidates others, adults must step in. It is not uncommon for children from 6 through 8 years to engage in this kind of behavior. However, adults must intervene in ways that allow all children to feel safe and comfortable at home or at school. Boys of this age who are continuing with their play themes of aggression and who are venturing as far as they can get from the adults may begin to intimidate girls or to make them feel uncomfortable. Although these actions are not the same as sexual harassment by adults and should not be treated in that way, when disregarded they teach both boys and girls to accept hostility and victimization.

Even though sexuality is a developmental function, humans learn the specific ways in which they behave sexually. To foster a safe environment, teachers must be aware of situations in which their response is required. Use of effective interpersonal communication techniques such as active listening provides support for children's development and leads to effective interventions that maintain a safe learning climate. Further, these strategies reduce the children's need for defensiveness and support their development of empathy (Ryan 2000).

Listen to what children are asking or saying. Be sure that you understand the meaning of a child's questions or comments. Wilson (1991) suggests some guidelines for adults when answering children's questions about sexuality:

• Find out more about the question by asking what the child already thinks or what she or he has already heard about the topic. Ask "What do *you* think about__?" or "What do you think__ means?"

• Check out the child's understanding both before and after answering his or her questions. After responding, ask the child to tell you his or her understanding of your response. Discuss further, if necessary, to ensure accuracy.

• Give honest information, and comment on your level of comfort with the content. Teachers and parents have different roles that lead to varying levels of comfort when responding to children's questions about sexuality. Values can be incorporated as long as they do not infringe on an honest response.

• Avoid technical language, but do use correct terms. Check to make sure that the child understands the meaning of the terms you use.

Addressing media influences on young children

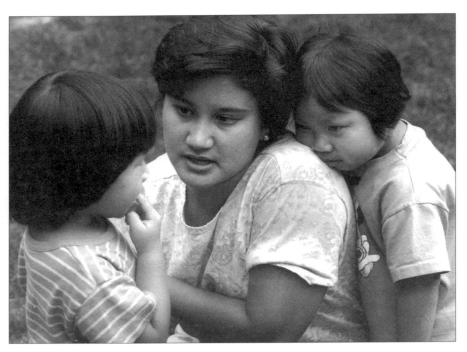

A great deal of concern has been expressed with respect to negative effects that television and other media have on young children. Much of this concern emphasizes children's exposure to media violence (Horton & Zimmer 1994; Slaby et al. 1995). We must also consider, however, the amount of sexual content in media productions that is accessible to children. Some of this sexual content is actually violent. Other sexual content may be either unrealistic or unhealthy.

In addition, another concern arises that is related to children's developmental levels and what is appropriate for them to view. When children view sexual violence such as rape in media productions, adults are unlikely to initiate discussions about it. Yet if children are viewing these kinds of interactions, they may then be affected in some of the same ways children are influenced by violence with other themes:

• Children may identify with the aggressor, and if they watch a lot of violence over time, they may engage in violent, criminal acts as adults (Huesmann et al. 1984; Comstock & Paik 1990).

• Children may identify with the victim and suffer from increased fear because they may believe that the violence is relevant to their own lives (Gerbner et al. 1978).

• Children may take on the bystander effect that leads to "increased callousness, desensitization, and behavioral indifference toward real-life violence among others" (Slaby et al. 1995, 166).

• Children who watch more violence are often more violent in real life (Liebert & Sprafkin 1988; Huston et al. 1992; Donnerstein, Slaby, & Eron

1994); this may happen with sexual violence as well and be carried over into play behavior.

Viewing media violence is likely to have different effects for individual children, depending in part on their developmental levels, temperament, and life experiences. One aspect of life experience that clearly influences these effects is gender. Violence with a sexual theme most likely shows males as aggressors and females as victims. Very young children who are learning about what it means to be a male and what it means to be a female are presented with extremely negative models in sexually violent shows (Hendrix & Slaby 1991). The concern that children may identify with these models is hard to overstate, and yet adults are not likely either to acknowledge what children have seen or to discuss it with them in any way that relates to a healthy reality.

Sexual content in television programming or in movies made for adult viewing is often not appropriate for children because of their different intellectual, social, and emotional levels of development. Adults are more capable of evaluating the sexual content that they view in light of their own experiences and values. In contrast, young children may attempt to incorporate what they view into their play in ways that may be inappropriate. Thus, guidelines for parents and other family members that provide information about viewing television and movies should explicitly recommend limiting this viewing and should suggest ways to discuss these situations with children.

In the article "Too Sexy Too Soon" Dianne Hales (2001, 44) includes the following guidelines for families:

• Keep TVs and computers in family space
• Don't assume anything goes over a child's head
• Don't encourage sexual precociousness
• Keep the conversation going

The information contained in this article could be included in a meeting with families, shared during a conference, or included in a newsletter.

Teaching respectful attitudes and behavior

With the increase of serious school violence in the past decade, many educators have begun to explore various models for peaceful conflict resolution. These models also might be used to address gender or sexual issues and behaviors that are aggressive or violent in nature. Teaching respect for all children includes the idea that we respect people who are different with respect to their culture, ethnicity, language, race, abilities, and gender. Sometimes, because of an immediate concern about a racial or cultural conflict, teachers minimize the effect that differences between boys and girls can have on children. Also, because of their own socialization, adults are sometimes insensitive to gender conflicts within the classroom or school.

When interactions between or among males and females in the classroom have sexual overtones, especially a combination of aggressive and sexual overtones, it makes sense for teachers to use a conflict resolution strategy. Any one of many conflict management models can be useful; however, children should use the same conflict management strategy for gender-related issues that they use for other conflicts in the classroom. Effective models achieve the following (Pirtle, as cited in Gartrell 1998):

• Children gain effective communication skills.

- Children learn that they have options and choices in conflict situations.
- Children learn to identify behaviors that will make the problem worse.
- Children learn active listening skills and ways to state their feelings.
- Children learn to try to find win-win situations.
- Children learn a concise mediation method that may be identified in steps through an acronym, for example, **POPS** for **P**ut the problem into words; consider **O**ptions; **P**ut out a possible solution; **S**imply do it.
- Children have opportunities to use the model frequently and consistently.

Working with families

Through family handbooks, newsletters, or other ways, teachers should inform family members that it is not uncommon for primary-age children to ask questions about or demonstrate an interest in sex. When educators and families understand that this interest is to be expected, they may have an easier time staying calm and responding in appropriate ways to children's questions or behavior.

As teachers build a learning community in their classrooms, they should involve families. Families can support classroom efforts and clarify behavioral expectations at school by encouraging respectful interaction in all relationships, including those with members of the opposite gender. To ensure effective support, teachers should provide some examples of ways children demonstrate respect and caring for one another.

Early childhood educators who have a school-sanctioned sexuality education curriculum may find it easier to work with families on these issues. Even without this kind of curriculum, however, teachers must inform children and families about what behaviors, interests, and concerns are typical of children at this age and provide appropriate ways to deal with them. It is important to demonstrate sensitivity and respect for cultural or family differences as they become apparent.

Teachers should always respond to the following behaviors

Behaviors
(as identified by the Kempe Center)

Sexual aggressiveness, both physical and verbal

Attempts to expose another's genitals

Sexually explicit conversations, graffiti, peeping, exposing, and interest in pornography

Preoccupation with masturbation, mutual or group masturbation (Ryan 2000)

Suggested Responses for the Teacher
(from the authors)

Say "It's my job to keep you safe. I cannot let you hurt another child and I will not let others hurt you."

Lead the child over to a private space in the room and explain that other people's genitals are not for showing.

Say "I won't let you hurt someone by embarrassing them."

Affirm the child's curiosity about bodies but explain that these behaviors or words may hurt or bother others.

Affirm that masturbation may feel good to the child but restate that it is both private and personal.

Note: In general, avoid extremely emotional reactions and do not use judgmental words. During conferences with families, do not judge the child's behavior or their actions as parents. Affirm their responsibility as parents and emphasize the need to plan together.

If any of these behaviors persist after intervention, plan together with families and make necessary referrals through school counselors, psychologists, social workers, or other appropriate resources. These may lead to professional development for all the staff.

Teachers should always intervene to correct these behaviors

Behaviors (as identified by The Kempe Center)	Suggested Teacher Responses (from the authors)
Touching another's genitals	State clearly that bodies are personal. Say "Children may not touch anyone else's genitals."
Degrading or humiliating with a sexual theme	Affirm that all bodies are good and explain that it hurts other people when they hear words about their bodies that are not kind.
Inducing fear through threats or force	Explain that it is the adults' job to try to keep everyone safe and that teachers will not allow children to threaten or harm other children.
Making sexually explicit proposals, including in writing	Explain that some words are too personal for children to use with other children. Contact families so that they can talk to their children about these incidents and explain that this behavior is not allowed.
Engaging in chronic peeping, conversations about sexual themes, graffiti, or showing interest in pornography	Stop the children's behavior. Contact family for a discussion. Describe what you are seeing and hearing at school and ask for information from home. Design a plan together and set another time to meet to assess the plan.
Demonstrating compulsive masturbation or masturbation with penetration	Contact the family for a discussion. Ask if the child has had a recent physical examination to determine or eliminate a physical reason. Decide on a course of action for both school and home. Set another meeting to assess the effectiveness of the plan.
Simulating intercourse with peers, dolls, and so on, with clothes on	Redirect activity to another area. If the behavior continues explain that intercourse is not for children and that it is private. If the behavior continues contact the family for a conference and describe the behaviors. Gather information about behaviors at home and then plan a strategy for school.

Be alert to these behaviors and attitudes

Teachers and caregivers need to be careful about their own attitudes and behaviors when dealing with primary-age children. Reacting positively to children's inquisitiveness remains important, and adults need to provide age-appropriate answers and guidance when questions arise. Teachers also need to observe children's behaviors and attitudes closely.

Caregivers may observe some of the behaviors listed on pages 66 and 67 in children younger than primary-age, and they should respond to them. At the same time, primary-age children are typically more aware that certain actions or body parts are considered private and have usually had the opportunity to learn that they are expected to treat their classmates with respect, physically and emotionally. Consequently, teachers should probably to take such behaviors somewhat more seriously when one of them occurs with a primary-grade child rather than a preschooler.

Caregivers should avoid sexist attitudes and behaviors and actively discourage children from gender-biased behaviors. As adults we frequently need to do some consciousness-raising of our own to recognize and get beyond our own sexist habits and assumptions, absorbed over years of socialization. Children need positive models as well as adult encouragement to go beyond stereotypic gender role assumptions (Derman-Sparks and the A.B.C. Task Force 1989). Use literature, role plays, guest speakers (for example, a woman who is a firefighter or a man who is a nurse) and other strategies to expose children to nonsexist roles and interactions.

✳   ✳   ✳

Primary-age children remain curious about ideas related to sexuality. They may have been silenced about their concerns at times because, so often, adults redirect or ignore their questions. Children internalize the notion that they should not be asking questions or making comments about sex. Yet, they are sometimes inundated with sexual content from media sources. Caring adults must be prepared to provide children with information and to serve as positive role models for developing healthy relationships.

Healthy Sexuality Development

5

Professional Development for Fostering Children's Healthy Sexuality Development

Early childhood teachers who were interviewed in focus groups (Couchenour et al. 1997) stated that they had no specific course content or training in understanding young children's sexual development. When asked whether they had taken child development courses, most stated that they had but the topics did not include healthy sexuality. Related topics such as physical and social-emotional development were included, but sexual development was omitted. All of the teachers interviewed stated that they had knowledge of child abuse and neglect.

Professional development for understanding healthy sexuality development is a neglected but important topic in teacher training. Pamela Wilson (1991) lists four requirements of teacher training for understanding sexuality development. Teachers should

• Explore their own values with respect to sexuality.

• Gain relevant knowledge about children's healthy sexuality development.

• Learn appropriate methods of answering children's sexual questions.

• Practice appropriate methods of answering children's sexual questions.

Professional development experiences must be carefully planned and carried out if they are to support early childhood teachers in their understanding and application of human sexuality development in young children. Please see the Resource section (p. 81) for a list of categorized resources to support comprehensive and ongoing training for teachers.

Professional development suggestions

Professional development became crucial when we found that most teachers in our interviews (Couchenour et al. 1997) had not had formal training or course work in promoting or understanding healthy sexuality development of children. Listed below are suggested topics for staff trainings that will help teachers to promote healthy sexuality development. Each topic section also outlines the purpose of the training, goals for the session, concepts to be highlighted, and additional resources.

STAFF DEVELOPMENT 1: Discuss typical child development benchmarks and include sexuality development as part of the content.

Purpose: To understand all areas of child development, including sexuality development

Goals:

• To gain specific knowledge about each area of child development

• To gain specific developmental knowledge about sexuality

• To understand healthy sexuality development as a part of the whole-child approach to early childhood education

Concepts to be highlighted:

• The relationship of physical, social-emotional, and cognitive development to sexuality development

• Typical behaviors, actions, and responses of young children that need to be understood in developmental context

Resources:

Haffner, D.W. 1999. *From diapers to dating: A parent's guide to raising sexually healthy children*. New York: Newmarket.

Lively, V., & E. Lively. 1991. *Sexual development of young children*. Albany, NY: Delmar.

Sexuality Information and Education Council of the United States (SIECUS) Early Childhood Task Force. 1998. *Right from the start: Guidelines for sexuality issues, birth to five years*. New York: SIECUS.

STAFF DEVELOPMENT 2: Discuss questions, issues, and concepts that relate to sexuality development. Invite knowledgeable professionals such as social workers, psychologists, counselors, or therapists to lead discussions among staff members.

Purpose: To support staff in increasing their levels of comfort with sexuality development content

Goals:

• To promote discussion about the importance of being prepared for children's sexuality questions or behaviors

• To be equipped to teach in age-appropriate ways and to consider all areas of children's development

Concepts to be highlighted:

• Awareness of the continuum of sexuality development that begins at birth

• Typical behaviors and concerns about sexuality development demonstrated by young children

Resources:

Cyprian, J. 1998. *Teaching human sexuality: A Guide for parents and other caregivers*. Washington, DC: Child Welfare League of America.

Sexuality Information and Education Council of the United States (SIECUS) National Guidelines Task Force. 1996. *Guidelines for comprehensive sexuality education: Grades K through 12*. 2d ed. New York: SIECUS.

STAFF DEVELOPMENT 3: Write, update, or review policy statements for the staff and parent handbooks that clearly specify the center's or school's guidelines for developing healthy sexuality in young children.

Purpose: To help staff incorporate information into staff and parent handbooks that indicates that early sexuality development is related to all areas of children's development: physical, cognitive, social, and emotional

Goals:

• To increase awareness of typical behaviors or questions young children have related to sexuality (prior to any behavioral or verbal display)

• To prepare and inform staff and parents of best practices that are developmentally appropriate

Concepts to be highlighted:

• Sexuality is about who we are and is not just a set of behaviors

• Many children are curious about sexuality, just as they are curious about most everything else they encounter

• Teachers and parents must work together to create appropriate responses for fostering healthy sexuality development in young children

• Healthy sexuality development can be a barrier to sexual abuse or harassment

Possible content to be considered for handbooks:

• Statements that note roles for early childhood educators in supporting healthy sexuality development in young children

• Statements about the encouragement of a variety of play opportunities for both boys and girls

• Stated strategies for responding to children's questions about reproduction

• Stated policies about viewing the family as the primary sexuality educator

• Stated policies about valuing and understanding diversity in family structures

Resources:

Couchenour, D., & K. Chrisman. 2000. *Families, schools, and communities: Together for young children.* Albany, NY: Delmar.

Cyprian, J. 1998. *Teaching human sexuality: A guide for parents and other caregivers*. Washington, DC: Child Welfare League of America.

Haffner, D.W. 1999. *From diapers to dating: A parent's guide to raising sexually healthy children*. New York: Newmarket.

STAFF DEVELOPMENT 4: Role-play scenes and practice reactions to situations, for example, appropriate reactions to masturbation at group times, children touching one another's genitalia in the dramatic play center, or use of slang, sexually oriented words that are demeaning to others.

Purpose: To practice or rehearse professional responses and reactions to sexual behaviors or verbal comments

Goals:

• To understand what is typical for the age group and how to respond to particular situations

• To understand what is atypical for the age group and how to respond to those situations

• To prepare for the unexpected

• To practice calm, supportive tones

Concepts to be highlighted:

• Aspects of sexuality related to physical development: bodily functions, body parts, pleasant sensations

• Reasons that children use sexual slang words that are demeaning of others and are inappropriate

• Importance of teacher intervention when children engage in aggressive acts with sexual content

Resources:

Cyprian, J. 1998. *Teaching human sexuality: A guide for parents and other caregivers*. Washington, DC: Child Welfare League of America.

Haffner, D.W. 1999. *From diapers to dating: A parent's guide to raising sexually healthy children*. New York, NY: Newmarket.

Packer, A.J. 1995. What to expect of your children's sexuality. *Child Magazine* (September): 60.

SIECUS National Guidelines Task Force. 1996. *Guidelines for comprehensive sexuality education: Grades K through 12*. 2d ed. New York: SIECUS.

STAFF DEVELOPMENT 5: Practice using anatomically correct language for body parts (especially if this practice is not typical at your school or center).

Purpose: To become familiar with and practice using anatomically correct language for body parts

Goals:

• To practice language to respond accurately to children's questions

• To practice language to respond to children's aggressive behavior or use of demeaning language

Concepts to be highlighted:

• Use of correct language helps children's understandings of their bodies; it eliminates some of the mystery and confusion.

• Words have power; when children need to use descriptive language, they are better equipped if they have heard correct words before.

• Even when adults know words, it is important to practice saying them. When adults can use anatomically correct language for body parts without hesitation or embarrassment, then children will feel more comfortable and supported in using this language too.

Resources:

Lively, V., & E. Lively. 1991. *Sexual development of young children*. Albany, NY: Delmar.

Wilson, P.M. 1991. *When sex is the subject: Attitudes and answers for young children*. Santa Cruz: CA: Network Publications.

STAFF DEVELOPMENT 6: Role-play conversations with families to discuss healthy sexuality development topics or situations. Include situations with family members who are frustrated, angry, or upset.

Purpose of the session: To practice responding to families about a sexuality-related situation

Goals of the session:

• To become comfortable with discussing sexuality development with adults

• To appreciate and understand that sexuality development may be controversial, sensitive, or embarrassing to some parents

• To practice active listening and effective conflict resolution strategies

Concepts to be highlighted:

• Sexuality development is part of human development

• Being able to explain children's sexuality development to families is an important professional ability

• Supporting families in their role as primary sexuality educators fosters children's healthy sexuality development

Resources:

Cyprian, J. 1998. *Teaching human sexuality: A guide for parents and other caregivers.* Washington, DC: Child Welfare League of America.

Morgan, E.L. 1989. Talking with parents when concerns come up. *Young Children* 44 (2): 52–56.

✳   ✳   ✳

Professional development is an important part of any quality early childhood program. The inclusion of current, useful, and relevant resources undergirds professional development. The suggestions and resources included in this chapter are designed to promote quality of care and practical knowledge.

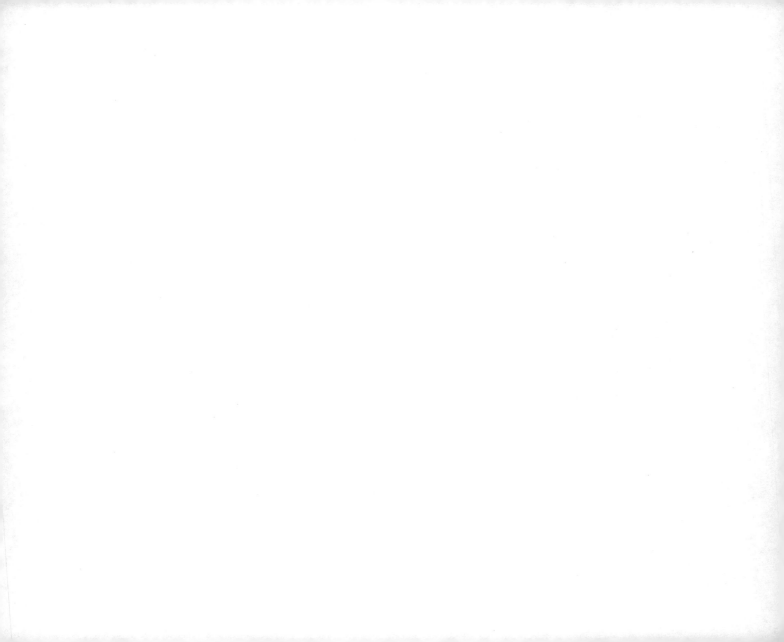

References

Ballan, M. 2001. Parents as sexuality educators for their children with developmental disabilities. *The SIECUS Report* 29 (3): 14–19.

Bredekamp, S., & C. Copple, eds. 1997. *Developmentally appropriate practice in early childhood programs*. Rev. ed. Washington, DC: NAEYC.

Briggs, D.C. 1970. *Your child's self-esteem*. Garden City, NY: Doubleday.

Comstock, G., & H. Paik. 1990. The effects of television violence on aggressive behavior; A metanalysis. Unpublished report to the National Academy of Science's Panel on the Understanding and Control of Violent Behavior, Washington, D.C.

Couchenour, D., & K. Chrisman. 2000a. *Families, schools, and communities: Together for young children*. Albany, NY: Delmar.

Couchenour, D., & K. Chrisman. 1996. Healthy sexuality development in young children. *Dimensions of Early Childhood* 24 (4): 30–36.

Couchenour, D., & K. Chrisman. 2000b. Healthy sexuality development in young children. In *Issues, advocacy and leadership in early education*, eds. M.A. Jensen & M.A. Hannibal, 22–27. Needham Heights, MA: Allyn & Bacon.

Couchenour, D., A. Gottshall, K. Chrisman, & T. Koons. 1997. Unpublished focus group interviews at NAEYC Annual Conference, 12–15 November, Anaheim, California.

Cyprian, J. 1998. *Teaching human sexuality: A guide for parents and other caregivers*. Washington, DC: Child Welfare League of America.

Derman-Sparks, L., & the A.B.C. Task Force. 1989. *Anti-bias curriculum: Tools for empowering young children*. Washington, DC: NAEYC.

Dispenza, M. 1999. *Our families, our children: The lesbian and gay child care task force report on quality child care*. Seattle, WA: The Lesbian and Gay Child Care

Task Force. Available online at www.safeschoolscoalition.org/ocof/ofoc_cover.html.

Donnerstein, E., R.G. Slaby, & L. Eron. 1994. The mass media and youth aggression. In *Reason to hope: a psychosocial perspective on violence and youth,* eds. L.D. Eron, J.H. Gentry, & P. Schlegel. Washington, DC: American Psychological Association.

Erikson, E.H. 1963. *Childhood and society.* 2d ed. New York: W.W. Norton.

Erikson, E.H. 1968. *Identity: Youth and crisis.* New York: W.W. Norton.

Field, T. 1998. Maternal depression effects on infants and early interventions. *Preventive Medicine* 17: 200–03.

Freud, S. 1917. *A general introduction to psychoanalysis.* New York: Washington Square Press.

Gartrell, D. 1998. *A guidance approach for the encouraging classroom.* 2d ed. Albany, NY: Delmar.

Gerbner, G., L. Gross, M. Jackson-Beeck, S. Jeffries-Fox, & N. Signorielli. 1978. Cultural indicators: Violence profile No. 9. *Journal of Communication* 28 (3): 176–207.

Greenspan, S.I. 1990. A developmental approach to pleasure and sexuality. In *Pleasure beyond the pleasure principle*, eds. R.A. Glick & S. Bone, 38–54. New Haven, CT: Yale University Press.

Hales, D. 2001. Too sexy too soon. *Parents* 76 (3): 92–94, 96, 98.

Hendrix, K., & R.G. Slaby. 1991. Cognitive mediation of television violence effects in adolescents. Paper pre-sented at the biennial meeting of the Society for Research in Child Development, 18–20 April, Seattle, Washington.

Honig, A.S. 2000. Psychosexual development in infants and young children. *Young Children* 55 (5): 70–77.

Horton, J., & J. Zimmer. 1994. *Media violence and children: A guide for parents.* Washington, DC: NAEYC.

Huesmann, L.R., L.D. Eron, M.M. Lefkowitz, & L.O. Walder. 1984. The stability of aggression over time and generations. *Developmental Psychology* 20: 1120–34.

Huston, A.C., E. Donnerstein, H. Fairchild, N.D. Feshbach, P. Katz, J.P. Murray, E.A. Rubinstein, B.L. Wilcox, & D. Auckerman. 1992. *Big world, small screen: The role of television in American society.* Lincoln: University of Nebraska Press.

Kostelnik, M.J., L.C. Stein, A.P. Whiren, & A.K. Soderman. 1998. *Guiding children's social development.* 3d ed. Albany, NY: Delmar.

Liebert, R.M., & J. Sprafkin. 1988. *The early window: Effects of television on children and youth.* 3d ed. New York: Pergamon.

Maccoby, E.E. 1998. *The two sexes: Growing up apart, coming together.* Cambridge, MA: Belknap.

Paley, V. 1981. *Wally's stories: Conversations in the kindergarten.* Cambridge, MA: Harvard University Press.

Piaget, J. [1936] 1952. *The origins of intelligence in children.* New York: International Universities Press.

M. Pietrzak, J. Heinz, A. Krugly, & D. Larson. 2000. Sexual orientation issues in the curriculum. Paper presented at the Association for Supervision and Curriculum Development's 55th Annual Conference, 25–27 March, New Orleans, Louisiana. Tape # 200088.

Rothbaum, F., A. Grauer, & D.J. Rubin. 1997. Becoming sexual: Differences between child and adult sexuality. *Young Children* 52 (6): 22–28.

Rubin, K.H., G.G. Fein, & B. Vandenberg. 1983. Play. In *Handbook of child psychology: Vol 4. Socialization, personality, and social development*, ed. E.M. Hetherington, P.H. Mussen, 693–774. New York: Wiley.

Ryan, G. 2000. Childhood sexuality: A decade of study. Part I—Research and curriculum development. *Child Abuse and Neglect* 24 (1): 33–48.

Santrock, J.W. 2001. *Child development.* 9th ed. New York: McGraw-Hill.

Schrank, L.W., & S. Hoke. 1998. *Raising sexually healthy children: Sexual development, sexual abuse prevention, and self-esteem for children under seven.* (Video.) Lake Zurich, IL: Learning Seed.

Slaby, R.G., W.C. Roedell, D. Arezzo, & K. Hendrix. 1995. *Early violence prevention: Tools for teachers of young children.* Washington, DC: NAEYC.

Schuhrke, B. 2000. Young children's curiosity about other people's genitals. *Journal of Psychology and Human Sexuality* 12 (1-2): 27–48.

SIECUS (Sexuality Information and Education Council of the United States) National Guidelines Task Force. 1996. *Guidelines for comprehensive sexuality education: Kindergarten–12th Grade.* 2d ed. New York: SIECUS.

SIECUS Early Childhood Task Force. 1998. *Right from the start: Guidelines for sexuality issues birth to five years.* New York: SIECUS.

Trawick-Smith, J. 1997. *Early childhood development: A multicultural perspective.* Upper Saddle River, NJ: Merrill.

Wardle, F. 1998. The expected and the dysfunctional: Dealing with child-to-child sexual behavior. *Early Childhood News* 16. Available online at www.EarlyChildhood.com/Articles/index.cfm?FuseAction=Article&A=120.

Wilson, P.M. 1991. *When sex is the subject: Attitudes and answers for young children.* Santa Cruz, CA: ETR Associates.

Resources

The following list of information resources is for families, teachers, and administrators to use individually or in groups. A section of resources for children is also included. Although some professional development resources for teachers and administrators are included in Chapter 5, many of the resources listed in this appendix will be useful as well. The resources here were chosen for both specific and broader, ongoing uses. Of course, each resource should be reviewed before use, and decisions should be made about its appropriateness for a specific audience.

Resources for children

Brooks, R. 1983. *So that's how I was born*. New York: Simon & Schuster.

Curtis, J.L. 1996. *Tell me again about the night I was born*. New York: HarperCollins.

Gee, R. 1991. *Babies: Understanding conception, birth and the first years*. London: Saffron Hill.

Gordon, S., & J. Gordon. 1992. *Did the sun shine before you were born? A sex education primer*. Amherst, NY: Prometheus.

Harris, R. 1999. *It's so amazing: A book about eggs, sperm, birth, babies, and families*. Cambridge, MA: Candlewick.

Jeunesse, G., & S. Perols (Translated by J. Riggs). 1995. *The human body*. New York: Scholastic.

Mayle, P. 1995. *Where did I come from? A guide for children and parents*. Secaucus, NJ: Lyle Stuart.

Mothers' Voices. 1998. *Finding our voices: Talking with our children about sexuality and AIDS*. New York: Author.

Newman, L. 1989. *Heather has two mommies*. Boston: Alyson.

Royston, A. 1996. *Where do babies come from?* New York: DK Publishing.

Schoen, M. 1990. *Bellybuttons are navels*. Buffalo, NY: Prometheus.

Whillock, S., & J. Norsworthy. 1992. *What's Inside? Baby*. New York: Dorling Kindersley.

Willhoite, M. 1991. *Daddy's roommate*. Boston: Alyson.

Resources for professionals and families

Periodicals

Professional journals and other periodicals provide a useful source of material for understanding young children's typical development. Listed below are some articles that both reflect current best practices and are useful for planning staff development.

Cahill, B.J., & R. Theilheimer. 1999. Can Tommy and Sam get married? Questions about gender, sexuality, and young children. *Young Children* 54 (1): 27–31.

Casper, V., H.K. Cuffaro, S. Schultz, J. Silin, & E. Wickens. 1996. Toward a most thorough understanding of the world: Sexual orientation and early childhood education. *Harvard Educational Review* 66 (2): 271–86.

Couchenour, D., & K. Chrisman. 1996. Healthy sexuality development in young children. *Dimensions of Early Childhood* 24 (4): 30–36.

Honig, A.S. 2000. Psychosexual development in infants and young children: Implications for caregivers. *Young Children* 55 (5): 70–77.

Katz, L.G. 1988. Those delicate questions about sex. *Parents Magazine* 63 (3): 162. Available online at http://npin.org/library/pre1998/n00355/n00355.html.

Katz, L.G. 1989. Nudity at home. *Parents Magazine* 64 (5): 208. Available online at http://npin.org/library/pre1998/n00192/n00192.html

Morgan, E.L. 1989. Talking with parents when concerns come up. *Young Children* 44 (2): 52–56.

Packer, A.J. 1995. What to expect of your children's sexuality. *Child Magazine* 10 (6): 60.

Rothbaum, F., A. Grauer, & D.J. Rubin. 1997. Becoming sexual: Differences between child and adult sexuality. *Young Children* 52 (6): 22–28.

Books and other resources

Books and other resources that contain useful information for teachers, administrators, and parents can be excellent materials for planning staff development. Listed below are recommended resources for designing workshops or training sessions, as well as useful children's books.

American Academy of Pediatrics. 1995. *Raising children to resist violence: What you can do.* Elk Grove Village, IL: Author.

American Psychological Association. 1992. *What makes kids care? Teaching gentleness in a violent world.* Washington, DC: Author.

Benstein, A.C. 1994. *Flight of the stork: What children think (and when) about sex and family building.* Indianapolis, IN: Perspectives Press.

Brick, P., N. Davis, M. Fischel, T. Lupo, A. MacVicar, & J. Marshall. 1989. *Bodies, birth and babies: Sexuality education in early childhood programs.* Hackensack, NJ: The Center for Family Life Education.

Casper, V., & S.B. Schultz. 1999. *Gay parents/straight schools.* New York: Teachers College Press.

Cyprian, J. 1998. *Teaching human sexuality: A guide for parents and other caregivers.* Washington, DC: Child Welfare League of America.

Derman-Sparks, L. & the A.B.C. Task Force. 1989. *Anti-bias curriculum: Tools for empowering young children.* Washington, DC: NAEYC.

Hickling, M. 1999. *More speaking of sex: What your children need to know and when they need to know it.* 2d ed. Kelowna, BC, Canada: Northstone.

Johnson, T.C. 1999. *Understanding your child's sexual behavior: What's natural and healthy.* Oakland, CA: New Harbinger.

Kreidler, W.J. 1994. *Teaching conflict resolution through children's literature.* New York, NY: Scholastic.

Levin, D.E. 1994. *Teaching young children in violent times: Building a peaceable classroom.* Cambridge, MA: Educators for Social Responsibility.

Lively, V., & E. Lively. 1991. *Sexual development of young children.* Albany, NY: Delmar.

NAEYC. 1996. *NAEYC position statement on violence in the lives of children.* Washington, DC: Author.

Pirtle, S. 1997. *Linking up: Building the peaceable classroom with music and movement.* Cambridge, MA: Educators for Social Responsibility.

Quackenbush, M., & S. Villarreal. 1992. *Does AIDS hurt? Educating young children about AIDS.* Santa Cruz, CA: ETR Associates.

Roffman, D.M. 2001. *Sex and sensibility: A parent's guide to talking sense about sex.* Cambridge, MA: Perseus.

Schwier, K.M., & D. Hingsburger. 2000. *Sexuality: Your sons and daughters with intellectual disability.* Baltimore, MD: Paul H. Brookes.

Sexuality Information and Education Council of the United States (SIECUS) Early Childhood Task Force. 1998. *Right from the start: Guidelines for sexuality issues birth to five years.* New York: SIECUS.

Wardle, F., ed. 1995. *Child-to-child sexual behavior in child care settings.* Golden, CO: Children's World Learning Centers.

Wilson, P.M. 1991. *When sex is the subject: Attitudes and answers for young children.* Santa Cruz, CA: Network.

Websites

Although the following Websites are primarily intended for parents, teachers and administrators can use them to help answer questions from parents or to support parents in their role as their children's most important sexuality educators. Most of the content would also be useful for preservice teachers in early childhood education, for staff training, or for individual study.

www.siecus.org/parent/index.html. From the Sexuality Information and Education Council of the U.S. Provides information for parents and other adults about sexuality education.

http://npin.org. The National Parent Information Network.

http://www.med.monash.edu.au/secasa/family/ html/child_development_sex_informat.html. Provides information about child development and sexual development.

Website articles

Haiken, B. 2002. *Toddler behavior: Masturbation.* Available online at www.BabyCenter.com/refcap/toddler/toddlerBehavior/11558.html.

Levin, D. 2002. *How to talk to your kids about sex in the media—Ages 5 to 8.* From BabyCenter.com. Available online at www.parentcenter.com/refcap/5554.html.

National PTA. 2002. *Talking with your child about sex.* Chicago, IL: Author. Available online at www.pta.org/parentinvolvement/healthsafety/hs_talking_sex.asp.

Planned Parenthood of East Central Illinois. 1999. *A look at the stages of sexual development from infancy to adulthood.* Champaign, IL: Author. Available online at http://npin.org/library/1999/n00125/n00125.html.

Sexuality Information and Education Council of the United States (SIECUS). *SIECUS Resources for parents: Radio Series: "Take A Minute to Talk About Sexuality with Your Kids."* Available online at www.siecus.org/parent/radio/radi0000.html.

VanClay, M. 2002. *Raising great kids: How to talk to your child about sex—Ages 3 to 4.* From BabyCenter.com. Available online at www.parentcenter.com/refcap/4388.html.

VanClay, M. 2002. *Raising great kids: How to talk to your child about sex—Age 5.* From BabyCenter.com. Available online at www.parentcenter.com/refcap/4394.html.

VanClay, M. 2002. *Raising great kids: How to talk to your child about sex—Ages 6 to 8.* From BabyCenter.com. Available online at www.parentcenter.com/refcap/4399.html.

Books about safe Internet access for children

For adults

Meers, T. 2000. *101 Best web sites for kids.* Lincolnwood, IL: Publications International.

Board on Children, Youth, and Families, National Research Council. 2001. *Nontechnical strategies to reduce children's exposure to inappropriate material on the Internet: Summary of workshop.* Washington, DC: National Academy Press.

Healthy Sexuality Development

For children

Cromwell, S. 1997. *My first book about the Internet.* Mahwah, NJ: Troll.

Videos

Bellybuttons are navels. 1985. Produced by Mark Schoen. 12 min.

Our whole lives (OWL): A lifespan sexuality education series. 1999. Produced by Unitarian Universalist Association and the United Church Board for Homeland Ministries.

> Our whole lives: Sexuality education for kindergarten through 1st grade. 8 sessions, 1 hour each. (parent guide available).

Plain talk for parents training package. 1997. Produced by Neighborhood House. Package includes video.

Raising healthy kids: Families talk about sexual health. Part 1. 1997. Produced by Family Health Productions. 30 min.

Raising sexually healthy children: Sexual development, sexual abuse prevention, and self-esteem for children under seven. 1998. Produced by Learning Seed. 25 min.

Sex: A topic for conversation with Dr. Sol Gordon, Program 1 (for parents of young children). 1987. Produced by Mandell Productions. 25 min.

Sex spelled out for parents. 1999. Series produced by Carson Street Productions.

> Sex spelled out for parents: Overview. 27 min.
>
> Sex spelled out for parents: Preschoolers. 27 min.
>
> Sex spelled out for parents: Primaries (Ages 5–8). 27 min.

Organizations

National PTA
330 North Wabash Avenue, Suite 2100
Chicago, IL 60611-3690
312-670-6782
800-307-4PTA (4782)
Fax: 312-670-6783
www.pta.org

SIECUS (Sexuality Information and Education Council of the United States)
130 West 42nd Street, Suite 350
New York, NY 10036
212-819-9770
Fax: 212-819-9776
e-mail: siecus@siecus.org
www.siecus.org

Early years are learning years

Become a member of NAEYC, and help make them count!

Just as you help young children learn and grow, the National Association for the Education of Young Children—your professional organization—supports you in the work you love. NAEYC is the world's largest early childhood education organization, with a national network of local, state, and regional Affiliates. We are more than 100,000 members working together to bring high-quality early learning opportunities to all children from birth through age eight.

Since 1926, NAEYC has provided educational services and resources for people working with children, including:

• *Young Children*, the award-winning journal (six issues a year) for early childhood educators

• **Books, posters, brochures, and videos** to support your work with young children and families

• **The NAEYC Annual Conference**, which brings tens of thousands of people together from across the country and around the world to share their expertise and ideas on the education of young children

• **Insurance plans** for members and programs

• **A voluntary accreditation system** to help programs reach national standards for high-quality early childhood education

• **Young Children International** to promote global communication and information exchanges

• **www.naeyc.org**—a dynamic Website with up-to-date information on all of our services and resources

To join NAEYC

To find a complete list of membership benefits and options or to join NAEYC online, visit **www.naeyc.org/membership.** Or you can mail this form to us.

(Membership must be for an individual, not a center or school.)

Name _____

Address_____

City_____ State_____ ZIP_____

E-mail _____

Phone (H)_____ (W)_____

❏ New member   ❏ Renewal ID # _____

Affiliate name/number _____

To determine your dues, you must visit **www.naeyc.org/membership** or call 800-424-2460, ext. 2002.

Indicate your payment option ❏ VISA   ❏ MasterCard

Card # _____Exp. date _____

Cardholder's name _____

Signature _____

Note: By joining NAEYC you also become a member of your state and local Affiliates.

Send this form and your payment to

NAEYC, PO Box 97156, Washington, DC 20090-7156